BIOBALANCE™

The Acid/Alkaline Solution to the Food-Mood-Health Puzzle

Dr. RUDOLF A. WILEY, PH.D.

Essential Science Publishing
Orem, Utah

Essential Science Publishing, Orem, Utah.

Made in the United States of America

First printing July 1989
Second printing October 1989
Third printing April 1990
Fourth printing August 1990
Fifth printing November 1998
Sixth printing October 2002

Library of Congress Cataloging in Publication Data

Wiley, Rudolf A., 1946-
    BioBalance: the acid/alkaline solution
    to the food mood-health puzzle

    Bibliography: p. 203
    1. Acid-base imbalances—Nutritional aspects—
Popular works. 2. Acid-base imbalances—Diet
therapy—Popular works. I. Title.

RC630.W55 1988   616.3'9   88-13740

ISBN 0-943685-05-2

Disclaimer

While it may be your constitutional right to implement the methods described in this book, it is suggested that you not undertake any diet, nutritional regimen or program of exercise without the direct supervision of a licensed and fully qualified physician.

DEDICATION

To Pam: there is nothing more admirable than when two people who
see eye to eye keep house as husband and wife, confounding their
enemies and delighting their friends, as they themselves know best.
(Homer, *The Odyssey,* (book VI)

To Jenni and Suzi and the world's children.

To the memory of George Watson, in hopes that his monumental
contribution will finally receive the recognition it deserves.

Table of Contents

Foreword

by Howard E. Hagglund, M.D.

Director, Hagglund Clinic (Norman, Oklahoma)
Member, American Academy of Environmental Medicine
Author, *Why Do I Feel So Bad When the Doctor Says I'm OK*

"FOR ANY SPECULATION WHICH DOES NOT AT FIRST GLANCE LOOK CRAZY, THERE IS NO HOPE" . . .

Freeman Dyson, Professor of Physics
Institute for Advanced Studies, Princeton, NJ

Stop! Reread that quote again. It will serve you well as you digest the importance of what Dr. Wiley has to say in this book.

In a busy, holistic practice, I spend hundreds of hours listening to patients. I am continually behind, and I believe I have heard as many reasons as to "Why I am sick and need your help, Doctor" as there are volumes in an encyclopedia. All usually goes quite comfortably until I hear this: "Doctor, I know this is all in my head. It's my nerves. I know it is all the stress that I am under." At this point, I become an absolute hawk... "not here, not in my practice. I won't put up with that kind of self-debasement until I am totally convinced that every physical possibility has been checked!" I have seen much success in treating patients for food allergies, candidiasis, and low thyroidism, etc. I should make this very clear to you now, reader, that I, too, am purposely biased in finding "the physical" causes of my patients' problems... this is why I think BioBalancing will be such a valuable tool, and I highly recommend it.

A few years back, I had the privilege of taking Dr. Tensley Harrison to dinner. We had a particular spot in Alabama in common. We were enjoying the memories of Alabama when our conversation turned to the Crock Award. Dr. Harrison would give this award to the first faculty member or resident that could prove a patient was sick for psychological reasons only. His only criterion was that he, himself, would be permitted to examine the patient and order the necessary laboratory test. If Dr. Harrison could not find something physically wrong, and then correct that patient's illness, this resident or faculty member would receive the Crock Award. NO ONE EVER CLAIMED THAT AWARD.

As practitioners read this book, each will find that there are patients whom they have helped by "their methods… where all others have failed miserably." I congratulate and praise all of you for that fine work. Now, as for those patients we have not helped – those we have dismissed as neurotic, hypochondriacal and "spineless"– this book… a gift… BioBalancing… is a great tool for their well being. Throw away your egos and those reflex criticisms. I feel we all know too little about nutrition and wellness to stand in the way of this book.

Preface

This book is the culmination of a 20 year effort involving more than 1000 individuals and the review of data on thousands more. The names of the characters in each case history are fictitious. Any resemblance to actual persons either living or deceased is purely coincidental. For the sake of brevity and for illustrative purposes, some case histories are composites drawn from several studies. This book represents my sincere desire to make available to the public information of momentous import which will, if given the attention it deserves by mainstream health care practitioners, revolutionize the way we view and treat both mental and physical disorders.

Early in my career as a physicist I was fascinated by what is known as the Mind/Body Problem — quantifying, or describing in scientific terms and according to the laws of physics, the link between the mind and the body. I felt that having studied physics to the master's level, I would seek an advanced degree in psychology in order to fully understand the connection between the physical world and the intriguing world of "the mind." However, my approach to the study of psychology was that of the trained scientist, i.e. to look for inconsistencies in methodology in order to discover why they existed and how they could be remedied. Much to my chagrin I found that there were numerous approaches to the study and treatment of mental disorders and none of them were consistent in their data. None could be statistically validated according to the methods I rigorously applied to them as I had been trained to do in my years of study of physics. I found that none of the dozens of labels given mental disorders could satisfactorily describe the underlying mechanism which creates the disorder so labeled. I wish to stress here that this conclusion was and is not now a personal opinion, but rather the result of applying the scientific approach, as it is taught in any field of science, to the study of psychology.

What I did next was again what any good scientist would do — look for another set of variables. Because I had, by a happy accident, stumbled upon the work of George Watson in the field of glucose oxidation and its effect on the psychological states of individuals, I chose to look at acid/alkaline biochemistry as it pertained to mental disorders. The results of my review of hundreds of patient records where plasma pH, a measure of the blood's acidity or alkalinity, was routinely done (but is no longer), revealed a strong correlation, one that deserved the attention of anyone truly committed to alleviating the suffering which I observed while studying and gathering my data in a state mental hospital. I was very excited by my findings, and being a young and enthusiastic idealist I was certain that as soon as I presented my data to the "powers that be" both in the university and the hospital administration, work in acid/alkaline biochemistry would commence and soon the doors of the hospital would fly open as the patients, now recovered, would issue forth in a great flood. At the very least I felt certain that I would be asked to conduct extensive research in the area of nutrition and its effect on mental disorders as the first step in opening those doors. My suggestion to the administrator, "Let's divide the patient population in half, you continue to treat your half by conventional methods — drugs, electroshock and "the talking cure," and I'll do nothing more for my half than change their diets!" No doubt I needn't tell you my data and my suggestion were poorly received by both the hospital and the university. I so shook up the establishment with my outrageous ideas regarding a link between food and mood that they chewed me up and spit me out, almost literally, not with the Ph.D. for which I had written my dissertation on the mind/body connection, but with a master's degree and a kick in the pants, here's your hat what's your hurry kind of exit. Those in psychology who had spent half their lives studying "relationships," refused to even consider the relationship between what we eat and what we feel.

After this debacle I spent the following few years working on my Ph.D. in biological physics, and continuing to mathematically articulate the relationship between biochemistry and psychophysiological function. I received my Ph.D. not uneventfully. It seems there was some confusion over whether my work should be judged by someone from the medical school, the department of mathematics, the biology department or the department of physics. Eventually this rather awkward problem was resolved and my Ph.D. was granted. However, I was no longer quite the idealist I had been, and although I considered medical school and in fact applied to several, I also realized that I had three strikes against me. I was already too old to be considered seriously by most medical schools, although constitutionally they were not at liberty to say so. Strike two — I had already spent several years bucking the establishment in psychology and physics. Medical school could only be worse. And the third strike was the climate in this country regarding health care at the time. Anyone exercising, taking vitamins and eating "healthful" foods on purpose was considered to be a "health nut," an expression you rarely hear today, but in the mid seventies was still prevalent. People were not yet ready or informed enough to begin taking responsibility for their own health and wellbeing. Physicians and psychiatrists were still the high priests of our society. And anyone outside of traditional mainstream medical care attempting to make waves was sure to get drowned.

Having come to this painful realization, I continued to gather and review data, and worked gratis with friends, acquaintances and referrals from those whom I had helped. Over the years the number of those helped continued to grow and this theory of acid/alkaline nutrition became fact. And then came the 80's and its emphasis on physical fitness, appearance and diet. Doctors began writing books on diets which they claimed could alleviate or cure various problems such as high cholesterol and heart disease, hyperactivity in children, premenstrual syndrome, and even stress and anxiety, two purely "mental" states now linked to food! How the world had changed in 20 or so years. Now dawned the age of the "holistic" M.D. and "alternative health care practitioners." And the phenomenal success of books on exercise and diet and the box office business being done by the holistic physician indicated to me that the time to introduce BioBalance Therapy to the public had finally come. The response of those seeking help through BioBalance Therapy and the success of those achieving a state of mental and physical health which had been denied them for years through traditional methods of health care was indeed gratifying.

However, this is not an overnight success story. Being a non-M.D. offering a health care service I was dogged again by the establishment and by the public mentality as well. No matter how dramatic and long-awaited the improvement in health experienced by my clients, the bottom line for a public long accustomed to being reimbursed for any and all health related services, regardless of the fact that they were frequently abysmal failures, was frequently, "Will I get reimbursed?" My clients all too often met with strong resistance from their health insurance companies. My work was not to receive the sanction of the multi billion dollar medical insurance industry. And most individuals found it very difficult, perhaps understandably so, to make even a modest financial commitment to this unknown, albeit highly successful approach to total health care.

So I now present my work to you, dear reader. It is my fondest hope that this book will break down the financial and political barriers which have prevented me from sharing BioBalance Therapy with you. We now live in a country where 75% to 90% of all patients seen by physicians suffer diffuse and undiagnosable symptoms. Some undergo extensive invasive testing. Some are given various drugs to reduce symptoms. Many are eventually referred for counseling or psychiatric "help." The physician has become lazy. He reads the printouts from the labs, sees the statement "within normal limits" (normal for whom?), believes it and sends his patient on to the psychiatrist. Next! Traditional medicine, a multi billion dollar industry, is failing as many as 3 out of 4 people in this country. And it's truly a crime. And often a crime of omission when you discover how many worthwhile, valuable theories and realities, such as BioBalance Therapy, are being ignored or viciously attacked by an establishment desperately determined to guard its territory. Medicine and psychiatry have shared the throne as "kings of the mountain" in this country and will not easily relinquish the stranglehold they have on us all.

I am asking that you judge this book and BioBalance Therapy, not on the basis of my credentials, or lack of them, but on the body of data which I present in as interesting and entertaining a fashion as I can in order for you to make an educated judgement as to the accuracy of my assertions regarding BioBalance. I know that if you do this you will find that what you are about to read is simply and profoundly the truth.

I

BioBalance Therapy Is For You

Every human being, regardless of his or her state of health, possesses some degree of acid/alkaline biochemical imbalance.

There are no exceptions to this rule. Therefore regardless of your state of health, you possess some degree of acid/alkaline biochemical imbalance.

Accordingly, this book was written for you!

Acid/alkaline biochemical imbalance is the culprit behind virtually all health related problems which commonly elude medical diagnosis, as well as many that do not. These problems are almost invariably misdiagnosed as "psychological," "psychosomatic," "stress related," "stress induced," "psychogenic," "attitudinal" or "mental." It is estimated that between 75% to 90% of all disorders which come to the attention of physicians are misdiagnosed in this fashion. If you are among the millions of people who possess a slight or moderate acid/alkaline imbalance you'll feel that you are "out of sorts," "under the weather" or "not feeling quite right" some of the time. If your occupation demands a great deal of responsibility, you already know that an imbalance resulting in this type of impaired performance is unacceptable since you will no longer be able to excel and be all that you can be despite your competence and level of effort. As any well trained athlete, astute corporate executive or skilled surgeon can tell you, at the crucial time, impairment of this nature can and will spell the difference between success and outright failure... failure that can result in the loss of a medal, the loss of a fortune or the loss of human life.

If you are among the tens of millions of people who possess chronic and severe acid/alkaline imbalances, your life has become a nightmare of endless and frustrating consultations with physicians who often refuse to believe your complaints, thinking that you are a *hypochondriac*. These well intentioned physicians might tell you that "everything is *within normal limits*," "nothing is physically wrong with you," "you're having a problem *coping with stress,"* "your problem seems to be of a psychological nature" and that "perhaps you should consult with a qualified psychotherapist."

Yet no matter how hard you try to follow through with your doctor's advice you just don't seem to get much better. Your symptoms may span a very broad spectrum encompassing (among dozens of other symptoms), fatigue, insomnia, headaches, body/backaches, inability to concentrate ("fuzzy headedness"/"cotton headedness"), anxiety-panic, premenstrual syndrome, digestion/elimination problems, abdominal "bloating" and weight management problems. You've probably also read countless books authored by the experts in alternative health care. You've spent a small fortune on vitamins, minerals and other assorted health aids, and you've patiently undergone treatment for such disorders as food allergies, hypoglycemia, candida (candidiasis), weak adrenals and (more recently) Epstein-Barr syndrome... without success. On the rebound from these demoralizing failures you wind up feeling guilty and go back to a psychotherapist thinking that perhaps your problem is of a "mental" nature after all. Your well intentioned psychotherapist is likely leading you to believe that your search for a solution outside of psychotherapy is an attempt to "escape" from the real problem which is somehow within you and which may require years (and another small fortune) to unravel.

The good news is that there is now a method of rapidly identifying, minimizing and ultimately eliminating your acid/alkaline biochemical imbalance. In so doing you can in turn eliminate your distress and achieve peak performance. The method of achieving peak performance as discussed in this book is known as *BioBalancing*. BioBalancing was developed after more than twenty years of careful research and application.

This book will show you:

> *why* modern medicine has failed in its attempt to treat many disorders which can be dealt with rapidly and successfully through the use of BioBalancing.

> *why* modern medicine has failed to understand how subtle changes in venous plasma pH, *the only valid measure of acid/alkaline imbalance,* are causing tens of millions of individuals varying degrees of distress which will invariably elude medical diagnosis.

why many *medically diagnosable* disorders lend themselves to BioBalancing and require far less (if any) medication than is conventionally administered.

why the practice of medicine without the use of BioBalancing is of necessity incomplete and is generally very far from complete.

why virtually all nutritional therapies discussed in the scientific literature and promoted in the popular literature fall short of the mark and *often backfire* by having you feel worse rather than better.

why psychotherapy is of extremely limited value and why psychotherapy does not offer benefits which surpass those derived from a good "heart-to-heart" talk with a confidant.

Perhaps more importantly, this book will show you:

how to identify your own set of acid/alkaline biochemical imbalances which make up your personal biochemical type known as a BioProfile.

how to use BioBalancing to eat in a fashion appropriate for your BioProfile and thereby reduce your imbalance and minimize the distress it is causing *for the rest of your life.*

how to evaluate *any book* about nutrition and health care in order to determine exactly who should and (more importantly) who should not be making use of the guidelines being proposed by that book's author. Such current "hot/runaway" best sellers such as *Fit for Life, Macrobiotics, Dr. Atkins' Super Energy Diet, Dr. Berger's Immune Power Diet, PMS: Premenstrual Syndrome, The Pritikin Promise, Psychodietetics* and *Eat to Win/Eat to Succeed* are only a few of the books which you will be taught to evaluate. You will also be shown which acid/alkaline biochemical types will benefit from the advice given by these books' authors and (more importantly) which biochemical types will suffer catastrophic metabolic damage by following through with their advice.

why your acid/alkaline biochemistry is the measure (without equal) which you must use in determining how you can achieve peak performance nutritionally, and why nutritional programs based upon other measures will only be successful through sheer luck, often hurting as many or more people than they would help.

why the maxim "one man's meat is another man's poison" is universally true within the context of BioBalancing, and why it is therefore *absurd* to classify nutritional regimens and supplements as being especially beneficial for (say) women with PMS, or women over 30, or joggers, or tennis players, or marathon runners, or football players, or highly stressed corporate executives, or individuals suffering from depression, or individuals suffering from anxiety, or individuals suffering from headaches… and the list goes on and on and on.

why some people *must* be vegetarians to achieve peak performance while others *must* eat red meat *daily* to achieve peak performance.

why the outcome of BioBalancing is not an "either or" situation; specifically, meat eaters need not fear that their new found feeling of well being and their ability to achieve peak performance must be traded off against a shortened life span and high risk of cardiovascular disease.

why the threat of elevated serum cholesterol may apply *only* to certain acid/alkaline biochemical types and not others.

why certain supplemental vitamins and minerals, even when taken in very pure or hypoallergenic form and in low to moderate dosages can be extremely destructive if taken by inappropriate biochemical types, irrespective of how "wholesome," "wonderful" or "safe" these supplements may be classified by the popular and scientific press.

why weight control has virtually nothing to do with "will power" and has almost everything to do with the degree of BioBalance you can achieve.

why eating in a fashion appropriate for your biochemical type
is easy and straightforward, and does not (as is the case with
misdiagnosed food allergies) require exotic, difficult to follow
menu plans.

While this book deals with nutrition and its impact upon human
health and behavior, this book is not yet another book about nutrition as
most people understand it. Instead, this book is about BioBalancing, a
revolutionary and successful approach in the understanding of human
health and behavior. As I've already stated, BioBalancing is not just for
the ill who are not receiving any satisfaction from the medical profession.

BIOBALANCING IS FOR EVERYONE!

BioBalancing allows you to optimize your psychological and
physiological well-being, irrespective of how you feel, and thereby lets
you biochemically truly be all that you can be.

BIOBALANCING IS FOR YOU!

II

What is BioBalance?

Panic attacks, migraine headaches, body aches, abdominal bloating and a losing battle to control her weight characterized Ann's condition. Even in her better moments Ann would experience unrelenting fatigue, an inability to focus her attention, all too frequent vaginal discharge and an ever present metallic taste in her mouth. She described her abdominal bloating as "the bloat," her inability to mentally focus as feeling "cotton headed" and "fuzzy headed" and her condition upon arising each morning as a feeling akin to having been "run over by a truck." Oftentimes she would go from one room to another in her house to get something and forget what she was trying to find. Ann's tragedy was compounded by the fact that she was 35 years of age and her symptoms had plagued her for more than 15 years. She had spent these years and tens of thousands of dollars on a variety of physicians who had repeatedly told her that all of her lab tests were "within normal limits," that there was "nothing physically wrong," she seemed to have "problems coping with stress," her problems seemed to be "psychological." In desperation she looked into alternative health care and underwent treatment for a variety of misdiagnosed disorders encompassing (among others), hypoglycemia, an overgrowth of yeast otherwise known as candidiasis, weak adrenals, pancreatitis, food allergies, and more recently a viral infestation called the Epstein-Barr Syndrome. She even had her amalgam tooth fillings replaced with gold when she was told that her problems resulted from mercury poisoning. She spent small fortunes and a restricted lifestyle pursuing treatments for each of these disorders. Nothing worked.

As a last resort she embarked upon a course of BioBalancing. At first she was predictably shocked by her recommended nutritional regimen consisting of red meat, fatty foods, and a reduced complex carbohydrate intake. The following is an example of her nutritional regimen during a typical day as outlined in her program of BioBalancing:

Breakfast: Sausages and eggs, well buttered toast, decaffeinated coffee with heavy cream.

Lunch: Mildly seasoned chili with a generous portion of chopped beef, buttered homefried potatoes, weak tea with half n' half.

Dinner: Sauteed liver, fried cauliflower, creamed spinach, herbal tea.

Ann's daily intake of supplements consisted *only* of the following vitamins and minerals and *none* other:

A, E, C, B12, inositol, choline, pantothenic acid, niacinamide, calcium, phosphorous, iodine and zinc.

As Ann stated it, "But this diet is exactly the *opposite* of how I've been eating." She knew that the regimen designed to put her into BioBalance was at odds with virtually all "modern day" conventional wisdom regarding nutrition and health. Her fear was further heightened by peer pressure from some of her friends who were vegetarian, macrobiotic or abstained from eating red meat. She was confronted with the usual warnings that eating in the fashion I've just described would place her at high risk for cardiovascular disease and would ultimately give her a stroke or kill her. One of her well intentioned friends who equated eating with social status and social consciousness went so far as to tell Ann that these nutritional recommendations were *"déclasse"* and just *"not California!"*

Yet her illness became so incapacitating that Ann was willing to try anything. Within one menstrual cycle after initiating her nutritional regimen she lost 15 pounds and felt significantly better. Within three menstrual cycles she achieved her ideal weight *for the first time in her adult life* and her symptoms vanished. She has not experienced a recurrence of symptoms within the past five years. Ann's triglyceride, cholesterol and low density lipid levels have incidentally also remained within normal limits during that period of time.

Melissa's medical history was not entirely different than Ann's with the exception that Melissa spent more than 10 years in *intensive* psychotherapy where she was told that she was suffering from "Post Traumatic Stress Disorder." Unlike Ann's nutritional regimen however, Melissa's regimen as recommended in her program of BioBalance Therapy was oriented closer to the lines of vegetarianism. Predictably, and unlike Ann, Melissa enthusiastically welcomed her nutritional recommendations since as she stated it, "This is just plain *wholesome* and *sensible* eating!" The following is an example of her nutritional regimen during a typical day as outlined in her program of BioBalancing:

Breakfast: Black coffee (not decaffeinated), 1/2 grapefruit, 1 glass of fresh squeezed orange juice spiked with fresh squeezed lemon juice.

Lunch: Low fat all natural yogurt (1% or skim) with pineapple chunks and mandarin orange slices; tossed salad consisting of fresh tomatoes, lettuce, radishes and onions with one teaspoon of safflower oil; black coffee (not decaffeinated).

Dinner: Poached filet of sole, brown rice, mustard greens, regular tea with lemon.

Melissa's daily intake of supplements consisted *only* of the following vitamins and minerals and *none* other:

B1, B2, B6, Niacin, C, D, Para Amino Benzoic Acid (PABA), magnesium, potassium, manganese, copper biotin, folic acid, chromium and iron.

Melissa's symptoms vanished within one week and have not recurred in three years.

Maria, yet another case, had symptoms which were remarkably similar to those exhibited by Ann and Melissa. Maria's nutritional *regimens* as prescribed by BioBalance Therapy consisted of a regimen similar to Ann's during the last 24 days within her menstrual cycle and a regimen similar to Melissa's during the first 4 days of her menstrual cycle. It is noteworthy that both Ann and Melissa each received different vitamin/mineral supplements even though in each case well intentioned physicians failed to identify any significant deficiencies through the use of blood tests, saliva tests, urine tests or hair analyses. As it turns out in each of these cases, popular wisdom claiming that all vitamin/mineral supplements taken "sensibly" and "in moderation" should be viewed as "insurance" and should therefore be regarded as good for everyone, simply did not apply.

As might be expected, Maria's supplements were similar to Ann's during the last 24 days of her cycle and similar to Melissa's during the first 4 days. Maria reported that prior to engaging in BioBalance Therapy, she had been taking a full spectrum, medium-potency vitamin/mineral supplement. Curiously, she reported that she had actually felt *better* on those days when she had *forgotten* to take her supplements. Given the fact that some components of her supplements actually *worked against her* during her cycle, it is easy to see why Maria responded poorly to her supplements. Since different subsets of a full spectrum supplement had to be "pulsed" to her during different phases of her menstrual cycle, Maria's observations are not at all surprising. Her physician, although well intentioned, thought Maria's remarks peculiar enough to recommend that she see a psychiatrist. Psychiatric treatment was the last thing that Maria needed.

Ann, Melissa, and Maria are only three of more than 1000 cases, approximately 90% of which have been successfully treated with BioBalancing. Why is it that three individuals who possessed remarkably similar symptoms were treated successfully in such radically different fashions? To understand the answer to this question it is necessary to answer the following question, "What is BioBalance?"

As any gardener or farmer can tell you, one of the first things you must do before you plant seeds or crops is to measure your soil's relative acidity or alkalinity. The measure of acid/alkaline balance of your soil is known as its *pH*. If you've done any gardening you'll know precisely what I'm talking about since you've probably taken pH measurements by looking at the color of dip sticks placed in your soil or by looking at the color of your soil after it has been placed in a prepared solution in a test tube. Typically, if that color becomes orange or red, the soil's pH is too low and it is too acidic. Conversely, if that color becomes somewhat blue, the soil's pH is too high and it is too alkaline. Some plants require relatively low pH soil which by definition is somewhat acidic. Other plants require relatively high pH soil which by definition is somewhat alkaline. Other plants require a relatively neutral environment. In summary then, the soil within which each species of plant or crop will be planted must be *pH balanced* for that particular species if the plants or crops in question are to be grown successfully. Any knowledgeable gardener or farmer would *never* invest money in nutrients, fungicides or pesticides for his or her plants or crops before first determining the acid/alkaline composition of the soil to be used. Investing in plant food or crop fertilizer, fungicides and pesticides is simply a waste of time and money if the application of these nutrients, fungicides and pesticides is carried out with disregard for the soil's acid/alkaline balance. This statement is true irrespective of how "wonderful," "wholesome," "sensible" or "organic" the plant/crop nutrients, fungicides and pesticides might be.

Simply stated, plants and crops grown in an environment which is either too acidic or too alkaline for the species in question will stand an excellent chance of succumbing to disease and parasites irrespective of how much "high quality" nutrition they are given.

Since one picture is worth a thousand words, the sketch presented below summarizes what I'm saying:

(Illustration 1.)

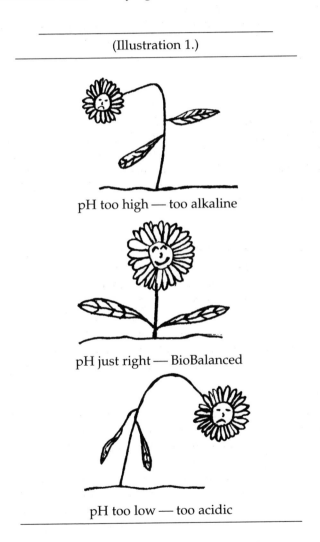

pH too high — too alkaline

pH just right — BioBalanced

pH too low — too acidic

The application of "common sense" in feeding plants and crops "wholesome" and "sensible" nutrients is clearly no guarantee that they will thrive if their soil is not biochemically balanced. Clearly, gardening and farming conducted with disregard for the soil's acid/alkaline biochemical balance will fall short of the mark. Indeed, the outcome of gardening and farming conducted in so irresponsible a fashion is by and large left to chance and sheer luck.

A strikingly similar situation applies to human health, be it physical or psychological. This similarity is in fact so strong that the following statements are perhaps the most important statements that I will make in this entire book.

THE PRACTICE OF MEDICINE AND PSYCHO-PHARMACOLOGY CONDUCTED WITH DISREGARD FOR BIOBALANCING MUST OF NECESSITY BE INCOMPLETE. THE OUTCOME OF THESE PRACTICES IN FAR TOO MANY CASES IS BY AND LARGE A MATTER OF SHEER LUCK.

Stop for a moment and think about the repercussions of what I just said. Imagine your shock if a physician told you that you were going to receive a blood transfusion and that neither your blood type nor the blood type of the donor was of any importance! A similar situation holds insofar as BioBalancing is concerned. After years of careful study, I can demonstrate that in many if not most cases, health care practitioners practicing medicine with disregard for BioBalancing are simply deluding themselves and their patients into believing they are getting "the best possible care."

What I am saying here is really the crux of this book and it will become increasingly clear to you as you read on. Furthermore, I will show you how you can personally determine your own biochemical type, (which I will refer to as a BioProfile) in order to achieve peak performance and improve the quality of your life.

As it turns out, *everybody* possesses some degree of acid/alkaline imbalance (or *BioImBalance* if you will) which can be minimized through the process of BioBalancing. The greater the imbalance, the greater the extent of your problem or "disease" which well intentioned physicians will invariably misdiagnose as "psychological," "stress related," "psychosomatic," "mental" or "attitudinal." These very same physicians will likely tell you that all of your biological indices are "within normal limits" and that there is "nothing physically wrong with you" and that "you should talk to a qualified (psycho)therapist." They might even think that you are a *hypochondriac*. I'll talk more about *hypochondriasis* later.

While knowledge of human biochemistry is not necessary to your understanding this book, a cursory discussion of human acid/alkaline biochemistry follows.

The type of pH to which I refer insofar as human health is concerned is called venous plasma pH, the measure of the relative acidity and alkalinity of the solid portion of the blood carried in your veins. This measure is as far as I can determine, the *only* accurate measure of overall human health because venous plasma pH registers molecular and ionic transfer occurring at your cellular level. While numerous books and treatises have been written about acid/alkaline biochemistry, with few exceptions none talk about venous plasma pH. Observations I have made over a twenty year period strongly point to the fact that other measures of acid/alkaline biochemistry including (among others) urine pH, fecal pH, arterial pH, saliva pH, sweat pH, toenail/fingernail pH, lachrymal or tear pH, hair pH and skin pH are simply *not* valid or complete indicators. *Only* venous plasma pH is a valid indicator since venous blood returns from your body's cellular sites of metabolic activity. Your venous blood's acid/alkaline balance therefore directly and precisely registers through molecular and ion transfer, how efficiently every cell throughout your body is converting nutrients into energy.

If what I've just said is unclear, then think of each cell in your body as a factory which converts nutrients into energy and creates waste in the process. Nutrients or fuel are carried to these factories in your arterial blood and waste is discharged into your venous blood. This nutrient-to-energy conversion process is critical in sustaining life and determines how efficiently your central nervous system will operate. Your central nervous system which includes your brain is a biological determinant of what is popularly called your *personality*.

Virtually all physicians I've spoken to don't understand BioBalancing because of the way "normal" venous plasma pH has been defined by the medical profession. Medically, normal pH is assigned a number value of 7.40. Don't worry about what this number means. I'll give you a feel for the acid/alkaline significance of pH in the next few pages of this book. It suffices to say that the lower the value of venous plasma pH, the more acidic the condition, while the higher the value, the more alkaline the condition. To add insult to injury, this medical definition's shortcomings are compounded by the fact that the medical community views "normal everyday" changes in venous plasma pH as inconsequential since these changes typically do not exceed one percent.

As it turns out, within the context of BioBalancing a value of venous plasma pH of 7.46 (*not* 7.40) is baseline normal and variations of 0.01 are extremely significant. Values of venous plasma pH substantially exceeding 7.46 point to an excessively alkaline condition, while values of pH substantially lower than 7.46 point to an excessively acidic condition. A variation of 0.01 over a range of 7.46 constitutes a variation ranging from one to two tenths of one percent. These differences often spell the difference between a healthy, motivated and well adjusted person, and a person who is tragically classified as "maladapted" and "neurotic" by the psychiatric establishment and condemned to a life of mental anguish.

Changes on the order of 0.01 are *not* insignificant as the medical profession generally concludes. An individual who displays an average pH in the immediate neighborhood of 7.49 is extremely alkaline while an individual whose pH is in the immediate neighborhood of 7.40 is extremely acidic. The highest and lowest values I've ever observed were 7.56 and 7.32 respectively. The two individuals whose biochemistries were characterized by these values were inmates in mental institutions. Both incidentally were released after they achieved BioBalance when their pH stabilized to an approximate value of 7.46. As you can see, in reality the medical definition of pH normalcy, a pH value of 7.40 equates to a state of *severe* acidosis!

Let's take another look at the cases I've already discussed.

Ann's venous plasma pH *averaged 7.39 over her entire menstrual cycle* prior to initiating BioBalance Therapy. Hence at that time Ann was extremely acidic. After completing her program of BioBalance Therapy, Ann's pH (again, averaged over her cycle) was 7.44, making her relatively normal.

Melissa on the other hand was extremely alkaline prior to initiating a program of BioBalance Therapy. When ill, Melissa's pH averaged 7.51 over her cycle. After experiencing complete symptom relief, Melissa's average pH hovered in the immediate neighborhood of 7.45.

Maria was extremely acidic during the last 24 days of her menstrual cycle and extremely alkaline during the first 4 days. When ill, Maria's pH averaged over the last 24 days of her cycle was 7.40, while her average pH averaged over the first 4 days of her cycle was 7.49. Maria's average pH was 7.46 during each of these phases after she had successfully completed a program of BioBalance Therapy.

The nutritional therapies which corrected the conditions which afflicted Ann, Melissa and Maria were very different in each case. The nutritional regimens recommended as part of BioBalance Therapy were not based upon symptoms, but were based rather on the type and the severity of the biochemical imbalance suffered by each of the individuals in question. By giving each of these women a different nutritional regimen, or as was the case with Maria, a *set* of nutritional *regimens*, the symptoms suffered by each of them were finally brought under control. To get a detailed description of the nutritional regimens used in each case you may wish to look at the Appendix.

It is noteworthy that in the cases described above, as in *all* cases of acid/alkaline disequilibrium or imbalance, disequilibrium is an expression of genetic makeup which articulates itself as impaired psychophysiological efficiency or "disease" as the result of nutritional intake inappropriate for a given biochemical type. I'll have more to say about genetics later. Hence **BioBalance is not a cure, but is instead a means of minimizing your imbalance and keeping it under** *control* **for as long as you adhere to your appropriate nutritional regimen(s).** Ann was made painfully aware of this fact when after being brought into BioBalance for several months she naively thought that she could "eat like a normal person" since she felt so well. Ann's definition of eating "like a normal person" meant eating in quasivegetarian fashion, a fashion she had adhered to prior to initiating her program of BioBalance Therapy. This style of eating accentuated the way in which Ann's genetic makeup was manifesting itself and was by and large contributing to her distress. Consequently, one week after deviating from her prescribed regimen, Ann's average venous plasma pH dropped to 7.41 and simultaneously (and not surprisingly) her symptoms returned.

The thrust of BioBalancing therefore consists of giving you a nutritional regimen appropriate for your acid/alkaline biochemical type *irrespective of your symptoms* and in so doing reducing or eliminating your acid/alkaline biochemical imbalance.

You will note that I said *a* nutritional regimen (or regimens) and not *the* appropriate nutritional regimen. It is critical to understand that there is no one nutritional regimen or diet appropriate for everyone. In fact, and as I've just implied, there isn't even one nutritional regimen appropriate for all individuals who display similar symptoms. The nutritional regimen appropriate for one extreme of the acid/alkaline spectrum, *irrespective of symptoms displayed by that extreme* is to some extent as you will see in the Appendix, the mirror image opposite of the regimen appropriate for the other extreme of that spectrum. So, even though two individuals may possess similar if not identical symptoms, BioBalancing determines what each individual's biochemical profile looks like before treating those individuals.

Individuals possess acid/alkaline biochemical BioProfiles... disorders which are routinely classified as "psychological," "psychosomatic," "psychogenic," "stress related," "mental" or "attitudinal" possess no such BioProfiles. If these statements lead you to wonder about the validity (or lack thereof) inherent in how the psychotherapeutic profession classifies so-called psychological disorders, you're already on the right track. I'll have considerably more to say about psychotherapy later in this book.

Just as each individual possesses a unique set of fingerprints or a unique signature, similarly each individual also possesses a personal acid/alkaline biochemical profile.

The case histories presented throughout this book should give you a good idea as to how BioBalancing can be effectively used in bringing under control problems which are commonly classified as psychological and thereby allow you to achieve peak performance.

Before continuing any further, it is well worth noting that BioBalancing offers a method of biochemical *control*. BioBalancing does not offer a cure. If you think of BioBalancing as being similar to taking a course of antibiotics, where you may eat as you please after achieving a state of BioBalance, then you are mistaken. Some individuals also mistakenly believe that while each person may be assigned a nutritional regimen which will correct a pre-existing acid/alkaline imbalance, each person should be assigned one universal diet directed at maintaining BioBalance once BioBalance has been achieved. Specifically, these individuals erroneously reason that once you achieve BioBalance, there exists one and only one nutritional regimen for everyone in a state of BioBalance. Observations based upon carefully controlled studies conducted over the past twenty years prove this belief to be incorrect. Oftentimes individuals who have formed a philosophic attachment to vegetarianism will state that while it is indeed possible that meat, fish and poultry may have temporary medicinal value, once a state of biochemical balance is achieved, only a variation of a vegetarian diet will sustain that balanced state. This is simply not the case.

Let me give you a good analogy which will serve to illustrate the truth of the matter and which should give you an idea as to how BioBalance Therapy figuratively works. Let's assume that individuals can be placed into any one of three categories, balloons or "floaters," stones or "sinkers," and "gliders." Let's assume further that in a room with an eight foot ceiling, a height of four feet above the floor is considered the ideal balance height. Left to their own devices, the floaters will escape equilibrium (the four foot balance height) by striking the ceiling. Left to their own devices, the sinkers will escape equilibrium by crashing to the floor. The gliders will without appropriate guidance occasionally hit the ceiling and may ultimately come dangerously close to crashing to the floor. How then can we cause any individual to achieve and maintain a state of equilibrium? By exerting a *continuous* downward force on the floaters, you will cause them to achieve and *maintain* their balance height. By exerting a *continuous* upward force on the sinkers, you will cause them to achieve and *maintain* their balance height. By exerting a *continuous* modified force on the gliders, biased somewhat in the upward direction you will cause them to achieve and *maintain* their balance height.

Given what I've already told you about venous plasma pH we can extend this analogy further. The sinkers are acidic types whose pH has a tendency to sink or decrease. The floaters are alkaline types whose pH has a tendency to rise or increase. The gliders are mixed or hybrid types resembling acidics in their tendency to sink somewhat more so than alkaline types. You will note that the key word I'm using here is the word *continuous*. If at any time you remove that force or substantially alter its direction, the floaters will rise, the sinkers will fall, and the gliders may start to pitch uncontrollably about a well defined flight path and may ultimately crash to the floor. Figuratively, this is precisely the situation insofar as BioBalancing is concerned. Acidic types eating in haphazard, random fashion will tend to gradually become more acidic. Alkaline types eating in haphazard, random fashion will gradually tend to become more alkaline. Mixed or hybrid types (which in the long term tend to resemble acidics more so than their alkaline counterparts) may start to deviate off course and may ultimately come dangerously close to spiraling into an uncontrolled dive.

The Appendix contains a detailed description of nutritional regimens appropriate for acidic, alkaline, and mixed types. The continuous *downward* force which alkaline types (floaters) will require to keep them from rising is a nutritional regimen which is therefore "acid inducing" in its potential. The continuous *upward* force which acidic types (sinkers) will require to keep them from falling is a nutritional regimen which is therefore "alkaline inducing" in its potential. The continuous force which mixed types (gliders) will require to keep them from deviating off course is a nutritional regimen which is mixed in its potential. Given the fact that mixed types tend to resemble acidic types somewhat more than they resemble alkaline types, their regimen must be somewhat more alkaline inducing in its potential than acid inducing. In fact, calorically the ratio of alkaline induction to acid induction in this case should be approximately 2:1. I'll give you examples of this regimen later.

The reason why some people are biochemically or metabolically designed to be floaters, while others are designed to be sinkers, while others are gliders is genetic. I'll explain in the next chapter that some individuals such as Maria are in fact genetically programmed to oscillate in well defined rhythms about the equilibrium level. While I will briefly touch upon genetics later, a detailed discussion of genetics and metabolism lies far beyond the scope of this book.

You should now understand why BioBalance is (as I've already stated) a means of control and why there is no one diet appropriate for everyone in BioBalance. The existence of only one diet appropriate for everyone in BioBalance would imply that somehow floaters and sinkers genetically transform into gliders when they achieve a state of equilibrium. Given the present state of the art, nutritionally induced genetic transformations of this nature are impossible to achieve.

III

The Crisis in Nutrition

It is fairly common to hear someone make the following statement, "I'm eating my yogurt, sprouts, salads, whole grains and organically grown poultry. I'm taking my vitamins and minerals daily… and I'm a wreck! I swear, sometimes I actually feel better if I forget to take my supplements. I'm becoming envious of my friends who eat whatever they want whenever they want it and feel pretty well most of the time. I've read all the *"in"* books on nutrition thinking that maybe if I take just one more vitamin or mineral or nutrient, then everything will come into focus and I'll be okay. But it never happens! Sometimes I feel like a vitamin and health food junky!"

It is easy to jump to conclusions and (erroneously) reason that in fact nutrition has little if anything to do with physical and emotional well-being and peak performance. After all, there are many very sick people with "undiagnosable illnesses" who are eternally trying some new type of diet and don't seem to improve, while there are also some very robust and hardy people who engage in haphazard eating practices and generally feel well. No doubt, almost anyone can point to an aunt, uncle, grandparent or great grandparent and claim that they ate whatever they wanted whenever they wanted it, drank liquor and smoked like fiends to boot, and lived disease free to a ripe old age only to die of natural causes. Doesn't that prove that nutrition has virtually nothing to do with good health? Doesn't that prove that it's all just a *state of mind*? I'll soon show you that such cases don't really prove much of anything other than the fact that some people are lucky in unwittingly and inadvertently locking on to a nutritional regimen or way of eating which is compatible with their biochemical type. Given the fact that you are reading this book, you can probably identify with the health conscious individual who is always ill or just not 100%. How do you account for this?

Physicians and psychiatrists will generally diagnose the health conscious individual whose health is not improving, if not deteriorating, as a *hypochondriac*. I always startle an audience when I state during a lecture that there is no such thing as a hypochondriac. I tell them that I believe *everything* that so-called hypochondriacs have to say. Do individuals go doctor shopping because they secretly, subconsciously or neurotically are looking for attention? I don't think so. People go doctor shopping because they are ill and want to get well.

Let's get back to the issue of why popular nutritional remedies outside of BioBalancing are by and large very limited in their effectiveness.

At this time there are numerous books and articles glutting the market trying to convince the public that each has THE ANSWER by way of *THE* DIET. While it would be presumptuous of me to claim to be an expert on all of the popular diets currently being promoted in the marketplace, the list below includes a few that have made it big and with which I have had firsthand experience:

> *Fit For Life*
> *The Feingold Diet*
> *The Pritikin Program*
> *The Dr. Berger Immune Power Diet*
> *The Dr. Randolph Allergen Free Rotation/Elimination Diet*
> *The Dr. Atkins Super Energy Diet*
> *Macrobiotics*
> *The Dr. Norris PMS Diet*
> *The Anti-Candida Diet*
> *Eat to Win/Eat to Succeed*
> *Psychodietetics*
> *How to Manage Your Mind and Mood Through Food*

I would suggest that you read these books carefully to obtain a better understanding of the ideas promoted in the 'How To/Self Care' marketplace so that you can form your opinion. I would also suggest that you read other books on nutrition and health as well since the implications of what I'm about to discuss are not confined to the books I list here. It is not my desire to misrepresent any of these books' authors. However, in my experience, each of these books (as in the case with so many others like them) reaches a major impasse. Each diet or program attempts to treat *you* without regard for your acid/alkaline biochemistry. Designing diets based upon your age, height, profession, sex, type of sport in which you participate... seldom works. You've already seen that identical supplements and nutrients can have radically different effects on individuals whose BioProfiles are radically different. For the sake of emphasis, let me repeat a previous statement. If a dietary regimen is devised with disregard for your acid/alkaline biochemistry then its effectiveness in assisting *you* is largely a matter of luck.

I have already shown that biochemical differences which should be gauged by acid/alkaline imbalances as quantified by venous plasma pH are extremely significant and typically make the decisive difference between optimal health and disease. To reiterate, while two individuals may manifest similar symptoms, there is no guarantee that their BioProfiles will be at all similar. Hence, it is sheer folly to prescribe nutritional remedies based upon symptoms alone. It is even greater folly to make *across-the-board* dietary recommendations to an entire population irrespective of variations in acid/alkaline biochemistry.

I generally find these across-the-board recommendations ludicrous while realizing the potential damage they can cause. Specifically some examples are (and I'm sure you've read or heard many more than I list here): less caffeine, less red meat, more vitamin B6 and evening primrose oil helps in controlling PMS; vitamin E helps in correcting impotence; B complex is good in fighting depression; B12 is helpful in combating fatigue; complex carbohydrates will help give you a "pick-me-up" while proteins will "soothe your nerves" (or vice versa); different classes of athletes should take different amino acids, etc.

Given the fact that you've come this far with this book you now understand why these across-the-board statements are either limited or, when taken together, are meaningless if not dangerous.

Perhaps the greatest nutritional threat to public health in general at this time is the medical/nutritional profession's media pitch for the *light diet*. Incidentally, with few exceptions, the *light diet* in one form or another is almost universally prescribed by today's nutrition gurus, irrespective of course of your acid/alkaline biochemical type. The *light diet* is one which has little if any red meat and is generally low in fat and cholesterol. This type of cuisine is currently viewed by many people as "wholesome and sensible eating." This diet is in many aspects similar to the diet appropriate for alkaline biochemical types. Hence, if you are not alkaline to begin with and if you self administer the light diet, the chances are excellent that you will feel awful in a short period of time. The author/ practitioner will of course cover himself/herself in this event by telling you that if you feel worse while "taking the (nutritional) cure" it's a good sign in that it means you're somehow discharging ugly toxins you have accumulated through years of poor nutrition and an inactive lifestyle. It should be clear to you at this point that if you feel worse and not better then the diet which the author in question has proposed for you (and everyone else) is inappropriate for your biochemical type.

Please note that I did not state that the *light diet* is universally bad. I did however state that the applicability of the light diet is limited in that if it is applied incorrectly it can make you feel worse and not better. Sadly, people have equated the *light diet* with an extension of youth and well-being and this mania for prolonged if not eternal youth and beauty has allowed the *light diet* to gain increased popularity. Advertising agencies have capitalized upon this mania and have convinced many individuals of the universal evil of such foods as red meat. To be slim, you are led to believe that eating 'light' will help, provided of course, that you exercise your "willpower" (more about willpower later).

To make matters worse, if you feel that low dietary fat is good, then less than low must be even better. If you truly believe this then you are in for a big surprise. By accentuating a dietary extreme such as the light diet, its applicability becomes more limited and it becomes more injurious to inappropriate biochemical types. Let me show you specifically what I am talking about.

Let's assume that your typical light diet (and there are many variations, each of which is not significant here), consists of poultry breasts (skinned), light meat fish, salad type vegetables, low fat dairy, whole grains and fresh fruit. Further, assume that dietary intake of fat is set at about 15% of the total number of calories. A dietary variant of this nature is applicable only to the extreme alkaline portion of any given population.

If you are either a biochemically mixed type, relatively acidic or oscillate in time, a diet of the nature which I am describing here can be harmful if not disastrous. The light diet which I describe is very acidifying in its potential, hence if you are relatively alkaline this acidifying potential will tend to neutralize your alkaline state and will result in your feeling well most of the time. If you possess a mixed biochemical profile, a diet of this nature can cause you to shift somewhat in the acid direction inducing a chronic acidic biochemical imbalance which will in turn produce problems which may manifest themselves behaviorally or psychologically or more generally prevent you from reaching your peak potential. If you are already suffering psychophysiological impairment because your biochemistry is too acidic, a diet of this nature can further accentuate your acid bio-chemical imbalance resulting in problems of a very serious nature which will likely incapacitate you. Individuals who are acidic will of course require a nutritional regimen similar to the regimen appropriate for acidic types (see the Appendix). This regimen is relatively high in specific classes of protein and consists as well of foods that are moderately rich in cholesterol and fat. This regimen is *only* appropriate for individuals who are acidic.

Indiscriminate application of *any* nutritional regimen will be equally dis-astrous in that it will accentuate pre-existing biochemical imbalances if applied to the inappropriate biochemical type. That is exactly why nutritional therapy when applied outside the context of BioBalancing is both very limited in its success rate and by and large does not work. If it works, it's the result of pure and simple luck... you have *inadvertently* locked onto a diet appro-priate for your biochemical type. Sadly, your new found well-being does not likely result from your conscious selection of the *optimal* regimen *for you*.

Put simply, I believe that biochemically you are not all that you can be until you have achieved BioBalance. Furthermore, your fortuitous new-found well-being certainly does not result from any insight that your diet's pro-moter had insofar as your biochemistry is concerned... you just lucked out!

Based on your understanding of what I have shared with you thus far, you will undoubtedly see that what is happening in the field of nutrition today is worrisome. There is a decided trend among dieticians and nutritionists to outdo each other in terms of giving out dietary advice which is biased in favor of lighter and lighter cuisine. Recognizing the imprudence of this trend, be prepared for a shock, because the situation is even worse than what I have thus far depicted.

I have only briefly touched upon the fact that your BioProfile is very likely inherited. Once again, genetics in the case of BioBalancing is not destiny, in that the manner in which your genetic makeup is expressing itself may be controlled through BioBalancing. I can tentatively conclude at this time that acidic genotypes among women are dominant over alkaline genotypes. Just as brown eyes seem to be genetically dominant over blue eyes, acid biochemical profiles among women seem to be dominant over alkaline biochemical profiles. Genetically therefore, future generations of women may *on average* tend to become more acidic. Thus, while the current popular fascination with the light diets is distressing, should this craze remain unchecked, it could have serious consequences in the future. It is reasonable to expect that "women's problems" such as PMS and "psychologically" related disorders will approach epidemic proportions should the light diet mania remain unchecked.

Today there is already a considerable fallout from these improper dietary recommendations. I will outline for you in the next chapter some representative case histories.

You may feel that I am being unnecessarily unkind to individuals who have authored popular books and articles on nutrition and health. I am not mean-spirited. My dissatisfaction results from the fact that there is a method which may *universally* be used in determining the efficacy of any nutritional therapy, or for that matter, any therapy. I discuss this methodology in detail in Chapter 10. Furthermore, I use this methodology in testing BioBalance Therapy.* In fact, this methodology is used in listing the relative efficacy of various diets as well as BioBalance Therapy. This listing is given at the end of this chapter.

The methodology to which I refer, known as the 'scientific technique', is more than 2500 years old. I clearly didn't invent it. The scientific technique should therefore be well known to most of the authors I deal with here (as it is to countless others). If these authors had bothered employing this methodology they would have seen the limitations of their nutritional therapies. Accordingly they should have honestly stated that their methods had limited validity, quantified that validity and cautioned that indiscriminate use of their diets could either cause harm or be valueless. This type of warning incidentally is not the same as a disclaimer telling you to see a doctor before trying out a diet. Disclaimers such as this serve only to minimize the author's and publisher's exposure to a lawsuit. Basing a self-help book on testimonial evidence alone is never satisfactory. People may be harmed as the result of an author's ignorance.

The list that follows entitled "A Consumer's Guide to Nutritional Therapy" gives you a preview of what lies ahead in the next chapter and simultaneously puts into perspective the realm of applicability of a set of nutritional programs currently receiving considerable public attention. The scientific method I briefly mentioned in this chapter and which is discussed in detail in chapter 10, was used to determine the success rate of each of the programs. You should realize that BioBalance Therapy is not a panacea. It is not a cure-all since approximately 10% of all individuals who engage in BioBalance Therapy derive no benefits whatsoever. Conversely, approximately 90% of individuals who have engaged in BioBalance Therapy report substantial benefits (ranging from substantial reduction in symptom intensity and frequency to complete recovery). Equally significant is the fact that when carried out in appropriate fashion, BioBalance Therapy should not make you sicker.

* as published in the *International Journal of Biosocial Research* (see references).

A CONSUMER'S GUIDE TO NUTRITIONAL THERAPY

Most books and articles on nutritional therapy are written with disregard for acid/alkaline biochemistry. Each author has unwittingly formulated a nutritional regimen appropriate for only one acid/alkaline biochemical type. Oftentimes these regimens are inappropriately administered. Such misapplication will invariably result in intensification of symptom severity regardless of how "wholesome," "well balanced," "sensible" or devoid of allergens that regimen may be. Subsequent deterioration of the patient's condition is frequently and erroneously misdiagnosed as some type of "discharge," "detoxification" or "healing crisis." In fact, misapplication or mismatching of this nature does not result in discharge but serves rather to accentuate a pre-existing acid/alkaline biochemical imbalance. Simply stated, a misapplication of a nutritional regimen can make you sick. If you are already sick, such a misapplication will have you out of the frying pan and into the fire by making you even sicker.

The following is a partial list of nutritional regimens currently receiving both popular and scholarly attention, and the acid/alkaline applicability of each regimen. Extremely acidic or alkaline states are represented by shifts in venous plasma pH of 1% from balance or set point pH. Moderately acidic/alkaline states are represented by shifts ranging from 0.5%, while mixed states are represented by shifts in the neighborhood of 0.1%. All of the individuals cited in Table 4.1 have made a sincere attempt at contributing to our efforts in understanding the role that diet plays in health. None should be faulted for failing to recognize the value of considering venous plasma pH measurements. I must reemphasize that it has taken me the better part of twenty years to establish its importance.

Table 4.1

Author	Regimen	Appropriate BioProfile/ *Success Rate (%)*
Rudolf A. Wiley, Ph.D.	BioBalancing	Individualized to accommodate all BioProfiles. *Success Rate equals 90% broken down as follows: a. complete recovery - 55% b. substantial improvement - 35% c. no improvement - 10%*

Table 4.1 continued

Author	Regimen	Appropriate BioProfile/ Success Rate (%)
Stuart Berger, M.D.	The Immune Power Diet	Moderately alkaline/25%
Richard Atkins, M.D.	The Super Energy Diet	Moderately acidic/25%
Ronald Norris, M.D.	The PMS Diet	Successful applications are primarily with alkaline types/25%
Ringsdorf & Cheraskin, M.D.	Psychodietetics	Variable but typically, extremely alkaline/25%
William Crook, M.D.	Anti-Candida regimen	Nominally acidic and mixed/10%
Orian Truss, M.D.	Anti-Candida regimen	Nominally acidic and mixed/10%
Benjamin Feingold, M.D.	Anti-Hyperkinesis Diet	Too varied and broad to permit evaluation/NA
Theron Randolph, M.D.	Allergen free elimination/ rotation diets	Too varied and broad to permit evaluation/NA
Judith Wurtman, Ph.D.	High complex carbohydrate diets	Extremely alkaline/25%
Michio Kushi	Macrobiotics	Moderately alkaline/25%
Nathan Pritikin	The Pritikin Program	Extremely alkaline/25%
Robert Haas, Ph.D.	Eat to Win/ Eat to Succeed	Extremely alkaline/ 25%
Harvey & Marilyn Diamond	Fit for Life	Extremely alkaline in the morning and moderately alkaline in the evening. The Fit for Life regimen is appropriate only for "diurnal cyclers"/10%

It cannot be too strongly emphasized that mismatching nutritional regimens will result in intensification of symptom severity. Hence nutritional therapy administered with disregard for any patient's acid/alkaline biochemical profile will typically fall short of the mark and may lead to adverse reactions.

As you can see, we have a considerable problem here. While no dietary therapy is a complete failure, the gap between the success of any dietary therapy and BioBalancing is quite substantial. I am not saying that each of the dietary therapies critiqued in this book (as well as countless others) is a total failure. What I am saying is that each of the therapies listed in this book is limited. I'll repeat what I said before, namely that random application of any dietary therapy without prior knowledge of your biochemical type is equivalent to playing nutritional Russian roulette, only here instead of loading one chamber of the gun's barrel and leaving the others empty, you load all of the chambers except one and fire away. Random application of dietary therapies will likely backfire and may cause you to feel quite ill or substantially worse. In essence, you may figuratively wind up blowing your metabolic brains out!

Phil Donahue hosted a forum about nutrition on his popular daytime television talk show where several authors/experts in the field of medicine and nutrition met for an hour and bickered with each other. In essence, each was telling the viewing audience that he was right and that the other fellow was a quack. I really thought this interaction was humorous, pathetic and quite illustrative of the sad state the fields of nutrition and health care are in today. The heated debate which I prefer calling a shouting match is reminiscent of the fable of the blind men and the elephant. If you are not familiar with this fable, let me recount it for you.

> It was six men of Indostan
> To learning much inclined,
> Who went to see the elephant
> Though all of them were blind,
> That each by observation
> Might satisfy his mind.
> The first approached the elephant,
> And happening to fall
> Against his broad and sturdy side,
> At once began to bawl:
> "Bless me! But the elephant
> Is very like a wall!"
> The second, feeling of the tusk,
> cried, "Ho! What have we here,

So very round and smooth and sharp?
"To me 'tis mighty clear
This wonder of an elephant
Is very like a spear!"
The third approached the animal
And happening to take
The squirming trunk within his hands,
Thus boldly up and spake:
"I see," quoth he, "the elephant
Is very like a snake!"
The fourth reached out his eager hand,
And felt about the knee.
"What most this wondrous beast is like
Is mighty plain," quoth he;
"'tis clear enough the elephant
Is very like a tree!"
The fifth, who chanced to touch the ear,
Said, "E'en the blindest man
Can tell what this resembles most;
Deny the fact who can,
This marvel of an elephant
Is very like a fan!"
The sixth no sooner had begun
About the beast to grope,
Than seizing on the swinging tail
That fell within his scope,
"I see," quoth he, "the elephant is very like a rope!"
And so these men of Indostan
Disputed loud and long,
Each in his own opinion,
Exceeding stiff and strong,
Though each was partly in the right
And all were in the wrong!

The nutritional elephant here is the acid/alkaline spectrum which I've already spoken about at length. Each *expert* espouses a diet appropriate for one portion of the spectrum and then goes on to apply sweeping and grandiose generalizations about the entire spectrum... "Everyone should eat only fruit in the morning!"..."Everyone should eat high protein meals!"..."Here's THE OPTIMAL DIET for everyone!"..."Everyone's diet should consist of approximately 55% brown rice!"..."There are no exceptions to my diet!"

If you reexamine my previous discussion of the acid/alkaline spectrum, you will see exactly how all of these dietary plans which I have discussed thus far fit together. While each is not completely inappropriate, each is limited in that it benefits only a specific biochemical type. If you are not that biochemical type, and if you have engaged in a particular diet inappropriate for you, that diet *must* of necessity backfire. The illustration which follows is a cartoon of the six blind men and the elephant. At this point the analogy between the blind men and the elephant on one hand and the *experts* and the acid/alkaline spectrum on the other hand should be quite clear.

(Illustration 2.)

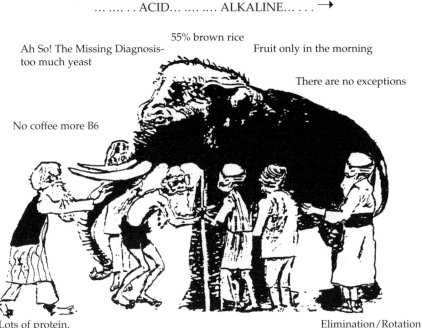

… …. . . ACID… …. …. ALKALINE… . . . →

55% brown rice

Ah So! The Missing Diagnosis-
too much yeast

Fruit only in the morning

There are no exceptions

No coffee more B6

Lots of protein,
Buffer your biochemistry!

Elimination/Rotation

LISTEN ONLY TO ME!

The Nutrition "Experts" are much like the blind men and the elephant…
although each is partly right, each is also wrong!

IV

Popular Nutritional Therapy: Life Histories

MACROBIOTICS

Macrobiotics may perhaps define one of the oldest sets of dietary laws in recorded history, possibly pre-dating Jewish kosher dietary laws. It would be impossible for me to do macrobiotics justice in so short a space. Its origins, dating back to ancient Japan, were largely influenced by Zen Buddhist philosophy. Macrobiotics classifies each food on a scale whose opposites are classified as Yin (yeen) and Yang (yang). Tomatoes, coffee, and eggplants provide some examples of extremely Yin foods. As it turns out, these foods also happen to be extremely acidifying or acid inducing. Eggs, meat and fish provide some examples of extremely Yang foods. As it turns out, these foods also happen to be extremely alkaline inducing. The pivotal point on the Yin/Yang scale lies in the neighborhood of the whole grains and is focused upon short grain brown rice. It is somewhat remarkable that there is considerable overlap between Yin and Yang on one hand and acid and alkaline on the other hand. This observation was made recently by one of the macrobiotic movement's leaders, Hermann Aihara, in his book *Acid/Alkaline*. It is however noteworthy that the similarities between acid/alkaline and Yin/Yang are limited. There are substantial contradictions. By way of example, bananas, avocados, asparagus, artichokes and spinach are considered to be rather Yin. As it turns out, these fruits and vegetables are not acid inducing but are instead alkaline inducing. As listed in the table given in the previous chapter, Macrobiotics provides nutritional regimens which are by and large acid inducing in their potential and are therefore only appropriate for alkaline types.

LIFE HISTORY: THE BIG MAC ATTACK

Sara was 38 years old. She described herself as a "baby-boomer" who had gone to college in the late 60's and early 70's, had witnessed and paid lip service to student activism, dabbled in mood altering drugs such as marijuana and LSD, had later married and had now become a young upwardly mobile urban professional or "yuppie" with a five year old child. Sara said she was a "hippie" turned "yuppie" and proud of it. She engaged in macrobiotics as a result of health problems which seemed to center around PMS (premenstrual syndrome) and which did not lend themselves to treatment via conventional and orthodox medical techniques. Her constellation of symptoms included severe migraine headaches just prior to her period as well as disabling cramps. Her other problems included a recent cessation of her menstrual cycle, vertigo accentuated by a prolapsed mitral valve, as well as fatigue. Her prolapsed mitral valve was symptomatic in that her heart would race and skip beats for no apparent reason. While these problems chronically plagued her, she stated that they got worse during the premenstrual phase of her cycle.

She had consulted with a macrobiotic advisor personally trained by Mishio Kushi, a leading practitioner of macrobiotics. Her advisor conducted a diagnosis including an analysis of her body type. Her large bone structure, olive complexion, black curly hair, and her physiognomy as well as her symptoms lead her advisor to tell Sara that she was excessively Yang and required a diet which would tilt to the Yin part of the Yin/Yang spectrum. She was told that her diet prior to engaging in macrobiotics was primarily responsible for her problem. Her premacrobiotic diet consisted primarily of *light* foods such as salads, light fish, poultry breast and low fat dairy. Approximately 15% of her caloric intake consisted of fat at that time. Diagnosed as too Yang, she was told to substantially reduce or ideally eliminate her intake of fish and dairy and to increase her intake of whole grains, especially brown rice. Her dietary intake of brown rice was set at approximately 50% of her caloric intake. The remainder of her diet consisted of Yin type vegetables and some fresh fruit which would be used to combat her Yang condition.

Sara immediately got worse. She was told this was a good sign in that she was discharging chemical toxins. Sara was very determined and held on. Peer pressure did not play an insignificant role. She attended macrobiotic cooking classes since macrobiotics places great emphasis on how food is prepared. In those classes, she reported, peer pressure continued to build.

An initial consultation revealed that Sara was not just hungry, she was chronically *starved*. She made her condition very clear, "I know that macrobiotics offers a very *clean* and *wholesome* cuisine, but I'm just never satisfied and I'm even putting on weight. Wow, I've gained 5 pounds! Nobody, and I mean nobody, gains weight on a macrobiotic diet!" She continued, "I would give my eyeteeth for a steak dinner, but my macrobiotic advisor says that's part of my western culture hang up. Lately though my symptoms have actually gotten far worse. I'm missing most of my menstrual periods, others are very irregular and the premenstrual syndrome has gotten worse too. I've become very irritable with my child and my husband. My husband keeps telling me I'm crazy and should just eat like a normal person. Believe me I'd like to. He eats red meat, has an occasional drink and even smokes once in a while and feels great! Can you believe that? And here I am being a virtuous macrobiotic person and feeling awful. My macrobiotic adviser tells me that feeling worse is not abnormal. I have to "discharge" my illness and that can be painful. Wow, I guess I'm paying for years of meat eating and for my ancestors' bad habits. What I can't figure out though is the fact that when I do have red meat – and I have cheated several times since becoming macrobiotic – I feel better. In fact, we went to a fast food restaurant where I had a hamburger with fries and my anxiety and depression lifted. Later I ate some barbecued pork ribs at a friend's picnic and I improved again. That stuff is bad for you, but I felt better! It must all be in my head because I still want meat so much."

Once again, while macrobiotics is beneficial for *some* individuals, it simply is not appropriate for many individuals, and Sara was certainly not one for whom macrobiotics was the answer. Given the fact that Sara was extremely acidic it was surprising to see that her macrobiotic diet had not inflicted more damage upon her than it had. When Sara received her nutritional guidelines in BioBalance Therapy, she was predictably amazed. Her response was typical, "I thought red meat was bad for *everyone*." Once again, it was explained to her that while fatty foods and red meat are injurious to some people, this was certainly not the case with everyone. She was also told that macrobiotics as well as her premacrobiotic eating habits (the "light diet") were primarily responsible for her problems.

"My husband is going to love BioBalancing," she responded, "he's always believed a good steak would help me overcome that washed out feeling I always get. My macrobiotic advisor will probably think this is crazy, but what the heck, if it works don't knock it." It worked very rapidly as it turns out. Over the next several weeks Sara lost 5 pounds and claimed she felt great. She was feeling much calmer and was experiencing higher levels of energy. Four months later, her menstrual cycle started up again, only now her premenstrual phase which had previously been quite painful was now almost painless except for a brief period of mild abdominal cramping at the onset of her menstruation. She was delighted. "My gynecologist can't believe my periods have started up again. She was ready to give me hormones. I told her about BioBalancing. She didn't say much. I also told the macrobiotic group about it. They told me I'd probably drop dead of a heart attack if I kept this up. I tried explaining this acid/alkaline, BioBalancing idea to them. All I got was resistance. One girl in our group got upset and said I was involved in fascist eating habits that would destroy the Third World. Wow, she really wants to lay a guilt trip on me. I just gave up. Well, here I am eating red meat and feeling great. And there they are eating macrobiotic foods and looking awful. I swear, sometimes I think life is really backwards."

This is an example of how Sara ate on a typical day while she engaged in Macrobiotics:

Breakfast: Weak barley miso soup with scallion bits (miso is a fermented grain paste), bancha twig tea.

Lunch: Tofu (bean curd) scrambled with a small amount of sesame seed oil and wakame (sea vegetable), mustard greens, long grain brown rice, bancha twig tea.

Dinner: Miso soup with shredded cucumber, short grain brown rice fashioned in nori (sea vegetable) role fashion with wasabi (Japanese horse radish), water sauteed broccoli and carrots, aduki beans with wakami, steamed apple or steamed pear, bancha twig tea.

Sara's average venous plasma pH while she adhered to macrobiotic eating practices was 7.41. This value is representative of a very acidic condition. If you recall, Sara had no menstrual cycle at that time so it is not appropriate to talk about menstrual cycle variations in her acid/alkaline biochemistry.

This rather picturesque and elegant fare gave way to the following cuisine after she engaged in BioBalance Therapy:

Breakfast: Small hamburger patty with fried egg, 1 thin slice of diet bread with peanut butter, 1 cup of decaffeinated tea with half n'half.

Lunch: Sardine sandwich (packed in olive oil) on thinly sliced diet bread with small amount of lettuce, celery and carrots, cup of herbal tea.

Dinner: Leg of lamb with gravy, brown rice with gravy and butter, spinach, herbal tea.

The supplements that Sara Took both during and after her program of BioBalance Therapy are listed in the Appendix in that section dealing with acidic biochemical types.

Sara's average pH after being brought into BioBalance is listed as follows:

average pH during her menstrual phase (days 1 through 4) = 7.47

average pH during her preovulatory phase (days 5 through 14) = 7.46

average pH during her premenstrual phase (days 15 through 28) = 7.44

FIT FOR LIFE

The Fit for Life program claims that getting well nutritionally is not so much a matter of what you eat but rather when and how you eat it. Nonetheless the program is very clear as to which foods should be eaten and which avoided. Some key dietary guidelines are summarized below:

1) Eat only fresh fruit and/or fresh squeezed fruit juice for breakfast between the hours of 4 am and 12 pm. Fruit is the most important food you can possibly eat.

2) Between noon and 8 pm eat foods in proper combinations. (The definition of proper combinations is given in the book *Fit For Life*.) Not only must foods be eaten in proper combinations but they should also be eaten sequentially described in the "energy ladder" scheme given as follows: fresh fruit and fruit juices; fresh vegetable juice and salads; steamed vegetables, raw nuts and seeds; grains, breads, potatoes, legumes; meat, chicken, fish, dairy.

3) Eat nothing between 8 pm and 4 am.

The guidelines provided by the authors of *Fit for Life* (Harvey and Marilyn Diamond) are clearly more complex than the simple guidelines mentioned here which are meant only to give you a summary glimpse of the Fit for Life approach. In order to take the guesswork out of the Fit for

Life program, Marilyn Diamond provides a menu in the book for the reader to follow. It should be obvious to you based upon the information which I have provided thus far, that the Fit for Life dietary approach is appropriate for only a select portion of the population and certainly does not apply to every individual (regardless of the claims made by the Diamonds). The case history below should give you a better idea of my concerns.

LIFE HISTORY: FAT AND FIT TO BE TIED

Gloria was 25 years old and described herself as "a nervous wreck." She was "eternally nervous and depressed." Her boyfriend Jack subscribed to the *Fit for Life* program as a means of dealing with a chronic lack of energy. As Gloria stated it, "Jack's transformation was awesome. He used to push himself to get things done and nap anytime he had the chance. Since trying the Fit for Life program, he just took off. He has energy to spare. He just raves about *Fit for Life*, wrote the Diamonds a letter thanking them, and got me hooked on the Fit for Life program too. The only trouble is that it didn't work for me. In fact, I actually got much worse. The book says I may get worse because of detoxification (sound familiar?). I don't know. I've been on the Fit of Life diet for about 8 months and if I detoxify any further I think I'll have to be committed to a mental institution. No kidding, as of last week it got so bad I started taking Valium. Jack says that maybe while his problem was biochemical, my problem may be more deep-rooted, you know – I'm *stressed out*, maybe I'm a *mental case* and maybe I ought to go see a shrink. All I know is that I'm about 20 pounds overweight and I feel like I could climb the walls." Gloria's fears were allayed when she was told that no one is really a "mental case." Her problem was not "mental" but rather stemmed from the fact that *Fit for Life* did not fit her. Jack's conclusions regarding Gloria are identical to the conclusions that your doctor may reach when his computer printout tells him that your bodily functions are all *within normal limits,* especially if you still persist in telling him that you just don't feel well. Hence he may conclude that your problems are stress related, you are having a tough time coping, you ought to see a psychiatrist. In summary, *Fit for Life* may have been appropriate for Jack but not for Gloria. In the acid/ alkaline scheme of things Jack was likely alkaline and accordingly capable of handling the *Fit for Life* regimen. Gloria clearly was not.

As is the case with virtually all diets being promoted in today's market, each diet has limited applications as is seen in this case with Jack and Gloria. *Fit for Life* can be applied with reasonable success to a subgroup of individuals who are alkaline during the early portion of the day and are only slightly alkaline in the late afternoon and early evening. Unknown to them, the Diamonds may possess these cyclic characteristics if they claim it benefits them. Unfortunately, the Diamonds have inadvertently generalized their experience to all individuals and have consequently developed a theory of cycles which they discuss in their book. The Diamonds' theory of cycles does not, of course, deal with acid/alkaline biochemistry. Not many individuals have acid/alkaline BioProfiles which mimic those possessed by the Diamonds. Static alkaline types whose biochemical profiles do not change appreciably throughout the day will do well on *Fit for Life* in the early morning then will not respond as favorably in the late afternoon and evening. Individuals whose biochemistry is of a mixed variety will not find the *Fit for Life* diet optimal and individuals who are acidic as was the case with Gloria, will find the diet absolutely intolerable.

Gloria's pH indicated that she was chronically in an acidic state which worsened a bit just prior to the onset of menstruation. *Fit for Life* accentuated her acidic state of biochemical imbalance. When Gloria was first given her nutritional recommendations as part of BioBalance Therapy she was horrified as are so many acidic types who have followed the popular allure of *eating light*.

"But the Diamonds say that fruit is the best food for everyone and now I'm told to eat heavy, meaty, greasy breakfasts. I'm sure Jack will think that this BioBalance stuff is a quack job. I just know that all that meat will putrefy in my intestines just like the Diamonds said it would. I don't know about all this. After all, the Diamonds said that we evolved from fruit eating ancestors and now I'm told to practically avoid fruit! Not only that, but if I eat this way I'll become a big fat blimp!"

Gloria was desperate enough to try anything, so she tried BioBalancing as a last resort. Jack carefully followed Gloria's progress and two months later was ecstatic over the fact that Gloria was transformed from a "neurotic fatso" into a "truly terrific and beautiful person." Gloria had stopped taking her Valium and had become, in Jack's words, "slim, mellow and really laid back." Gloria had also stated that her gastrointestinal problems, which had chronically plagued her, had all but vanished; her flatulence was gone and she was no longer constipated. She also reported having finally lost 19 pounds thereby achieving her ideal weight.

Unfortunately Gloria did have one major problem which she did not have before. That problem was Jack. Seeing the results of Gloria's regimen, Jack decided to try it. His response was immediate and cata-strophic. As he stated, "My depression and lack of energy came back in spades, but I must be detoxifying or something just like the Diamonds said in their book and I know when I get through this, the diet that worked for Gloria will work for me too." Nothing could have been further from the truth. The principles of BioBalancing had to be explained to both Jack and Gloria stressing the fact that while Gloria's diet was appropriate for her it was not appropriate for Jack. It turned out that Jack was so alkaline that a vegetarian diet, which to a great extent was a variation of the *Fit for Life* diet was recommended. Jack and Gloria both completed their program in BioBalancing soon thereafter, each claiming to be doing very well.

This is an example of how Gloria ate on a typical day while she engaged in the *Fit for Life* program. Once again, Jack thrived on this *identical* program:

Breakfast: Fresh squeezed orange juice with pulp, watermelon and casaba melon.

Lunch: All natural fruit juice followed by vegetable juice in a carrot base (home made in blender), steamed vegetables with rice cakes.

Dinner: Vegetable juice (same as lunch), fresh garden salad with "all natural," low salt, low fat dressing, steamed brown rice and millet with lentils and kale.

Gloria's pH while she was engaged in the *Fit for Life* regimen was:

average menstrual pH (days 1 through 4) = 7.42

average preovulatory pH (days 5 through 14) = 7.42

average premenstrual pH (days 15 through 28) = 7.40

This is an example of how Gloria ate on a typical day after she achieved BioBalance:

Breakfast: Bacon (preferably nitrate/nitrite free) and egg(s) (any style), herbal tea.

Lunch: Cup of lentil and beef soup, salmon salad (with mayonnaise, celery and carrots) stuffed in half an avocado, herbal tea.

Snack: Diet rye or wheat thins with peanut butter.

Dinner: Prime rib, buttered baked potato with buttered lima beans.

Gloria's pH after she achieved BioBalance was:

average menstrual pH (days 1 through 4) = 7.46

average preovulatory pH (days 5 through 14) = 7.45

average premenstrual pH (days 15 through 28) = 7.44

The supplements Gloria took during and after her program of BioBalance Therapy are listed in the Appendix in that section dealing with acidic biochemical types.

THE PRITIKIN PROGRAM

Nathan Pritikin offers a number of dietary guidelines in his book, *The Pritikin Promise*. The Pritikin Diet is ideally free of meat, at best treats meat as a condiment and stresses an increased intake of complex carbohydrates found in whole grains, fruits and vegetables. Furthermore, Pritikin believes that the ideal diet should have no added fat. According to Pritikin, the ideal diet will consist of 5% to 10% fat, 10% to 15% protein, and 80% complex carbohydrates. The small amount of meat included in the diet should be skinned white meat poultry or light fish. Pritikin emphasizes that meat is to be avoided if possible and points out that there is no such thing as superior and inferior protein. In support of this belief that meat is eaten in too great a quantity by industrialized societies, Pritikin points out that the Tarahumara Indians possess remarkably strong constitutions and are capable of remarkable physical activity despite the fact that they eat meat no more than several times a year. The Pritikin Program has been put together after years of careful thought and observation and primarily in response to the increased incidence of cardiovascular and coronary disease occurring throughout industrialized societies. The following case study will illustrate the limitations of the Pritikin Program.

LIFE HISTORY: HOW I STOPPED WORRYING AND LEARNED TO LOVE FILET MIGNON

Wayne was a 40 year-old business executive who felt that he was becoming too easily fatigued and was losing his war against obesity despite his strenuous daily workout. Accordingly, he decided to spend his vacation at a health resort which employed dietary practices similar to those developed by Nathan Pritikin.

"I've spent most of my life fighting the battle of the bulge," Wayne stated amicably pointing to his belly. "My dad was a diabetic and I saw him die a gruesome death. I decided to take charge of my health. I've never trusted doctors. All they're equipped to do is give you medication to get rid of your symptoms, but I don't think they ever get to the real problem. I've been working out for the past six years and I watch my diet. I've read a good deal about nutrition and I must say that Pritikin's book really impressed me. I decided to take the plunge and sign up at a health and fitness center using Pritikin's techniques. I must confess that I was quite impressed with the operation. I just can't believe I felt so awful during my stay. My malaise was compounded by the fact that everyone around me was doing so well, or at least it seemed that way to me. I got more and more tired and very hungry. I swear, I could have eaten a large steak, fat and all, if I'd had the chance! But I know that stuff is murder and no way am I going to wind up like my dad. By sheer force of will I just dragged myself along. After a while my hunger just turned to nausea and the smell of food disgusted me. By this time I was having weird dream fragments every night just before I feel asleep. I think they're called eidetic images — some really scary. Then I started getting nervous, so I finally couldn't sleep at all. This would make a great report, *What I Did For My Summer Vacation,* or even better I should write a book and get the movie rights!" Wayne laughed. "When I asked about my insomnia, I was told to relax. I was told that I worried too much. I asked if maybe I should try a different diet, and was told that there is *no* exception to the Pritikin Diet. When my stay at the center ended, I dragged myself out and wolfed down a steak. I swear I felt better for a couple of hours. That's why I want to try BioBalancing. All these diets are just too confusing. I give up!"

Wayne appeared to be a mixed type with a tendency to "spike" acidic on occasion. His acidic state was accentuated, no doubt, by his stay at the health and fitness center where his diet was more appropriate for very alkaline biochemical types. Wayne was somewhat relieved when he was given his dietary recommendations. "Wow! This just sounds just too good to be true. Steak, liver, eggs, fried potatoes. I love these foods. What about my health? I have a vision of myself dying like my dad."

Wayne was told that his dad was diabetic and therefore probably possessed a biochemical type opposite that of Wayne's. As I've already stated, your BioProfile is not inherited in a straightforward linear fashion. As is the case with eye color, it is possible for parents to genetically transmit BioProfiles to their children which are radically different than their own. This should not surprise you since few traits are inherited in simple fashion. To repeat, it is possible for two brown eyed parents to give birth to blue eyed children. Similarly it is possible for an alkaline male to be the biological father of an acidic child. Genetic factors incidentally, likely offer an explanation as to why the Tarahumara Indians which Pritikin points to, do so well on a diet rich in complex carbohydrates and conspicuously absent of meat. I would speculate that the Tarahumaras are relatively alkaline. It is also my guess that by inbreeding, the alkaline trait survived since any acidic Tarahumaras became quite badly impaired and maladapted and died as a result of their rigorous life style. This entire process is known as natural selection.

Wayne did very well in BioBalance Therapy. During his follow up consultation he reported feeling great. "I feel energized. I go to work feeling clear headed. I feel rejuvenated after working out at the health spa. I'm also sleeping well again. Imagine being made to feel guilty by being told that I worry too much. Well, I guess another fad diet bites the dust. Poor old departed Pritikin."

It is true as Wayne intimated that the Pritikin Program was limited in its approach, although admittedly quite effective in dealing with specific alkaline types. However, Wayne was also led to understand that one cannot evaluate a nutritional therapy on the basis of the health or lack of health of its founder. Sadly and not infrequently, the author of a book will promote that book based on the fact that he or she used certain techniques to lose an enormous amount of weight, or outlive the competition, or snatch some celebrity from death's door, etc. As I've already implied, this appeal to high drama is completely irrelevant insofar as the efficacy of any treatment methodology (nutritional or otherwise) is concerned. The efficacy of any therapy can only be evaluated in terms of its success in dealing with a large population. The success of any therapy should *never* be judged on the basis of the health of its founder. Should we scrap the polio vaccine if Jonas Salk, its developer, is found crippled with polio? Although I can only speculate regarding the biochemical type of the originator or proponents of any given dietary program, I judge its efficacy solely by the percentage of people successfully treated. As I already mentioned, I'll show you in Chapter 10 how to rapidly evaluate *any* given therapy.

This is an example of how Wayne ate on a typical day when he was involved the Pritikin program:

Breakfast: Skim yogurt with fresh fruit and all natural sugar free whole grain cereal, herbal tea.

Lunch: Mock cream of potato soup (with skim milk and stone ground wheat flour as a "cream" base), steamed squash with beans, brown rice cakes, vegetable juice.

Dinner: Small portion of flounder filet (poached), steamed buckwheat and broccoli with low salt, zero fat tomato sauce (home made), herbal tea.

Wayne's average venous plasma pH while engaging in the Pritikin program was 7.43.

This is an example of how Wayne ate on a typical day during and after engaging in BioBalance Therapy:

Breakfast: Glass of apple juice, cup of whole oats with 2% milk, whole grain bread with nut butter (any variety), decaffeinated tea.

Lunch: Cup of vegetarian style chili, chicken salad sandwich on whole grain bread with light and dark meat chicken and mayonnaise, celery and onions, glass of all natural fruit punch.

Dinner: Stir fry containing salmon, shrimp and flounder with brown rice, onions, carrots, cauliflower and broccoli, glass of decaffeinated tea.

If you look at the other regimens I've listed thus far you will note that Wayne's regimen is a good example of the fact that mixed types should eat in a fashion which mixes foods appropriate for both acidic types and alkaline types, relying a bit more on those foods appropriate for acidic types. The reason for this bias stems from the fact that it is easier for a mixed type to become excessively acidic than to become excessively alkaline. A good rule of thumb for mixed types to follow is to mix the regimens appropriate for acidic and alkaline types in a caloric ratio of 2:1 in favor of the regimen appropriate for acidics. Acidic types *must* on the other hand avoid all foods appropriate for alkaline types (and vice versa). Acidic types must also eat their meats, fish and poultry at *every* meal. Mixed types may on occasion abstain from meat, fish or poultry during breakfast, but they *must* eat the appropriate admixture (2:1) of meat, fish or poultry for both lunch and dinner.

The supplements Wayne took are described in the Appendix under "mixed types."

Wayne's average pH after achieving BioBalance was 7.47.

THE DR. ATKINS SUPER ENERGY DIET

Amid all the *light diets* the Dr. Atkins Super Energy Diet probably stands alone. Dr. Atkins bases his dietary therapy upon the successful treatment of hypoglycemia and as such he recognizes the need for a diet rich in protein and moderate in fat. The word hypoglycemia evolves from the Latin, "hypo" meaning low and "glycemia" meaning sugar. Individuals who are hypoglycemic generally possess low levels of fasting blood sugar. Dr. Atkins has had clinical success in dealing with hypoglycemia. He believes that many patients who present their physicians with a long list of complaints and whose ailments are generally "undiagnosable" are probably hypoglycemic. This belief is partially correct.

Let's go back to the acid/alkaline spectrum I discussed in Chapter 2 to see why Dr. Atkins is only partially correct. It turns out that acidic types generally tend to burn up blood sugar or glucose faster than alkaline or mixed types. Hence, the more acidic the biochemical type, the more rapid the rate at which blood sugar is being consumed. Therefore, individuals who populate the extreme acid end of the acid/alkaline spectrum tend to burn up blood sugar very rapidly and are by definition *extreme hypoglycemics*. Those who fall on the acid side of normal but who are not extremely acidic are only mildly hypoglycemic.

The measure Dr. Atkins uses in determining hypoglycemia is the glucose tolerance test. This test is administered by giving the patient an oral dose of glucola (a sugar solution) and then drawing the patient's blood every half hour to one hour within a period of time ranging from 4 to 7 hours after the ingestion of the glucola. Each blood sample is then analyzed to determine the blood sugar concentration at a particular time.

As it turns out, the glucose tolerance curve is a limited indicator of an underlying metabolic or biochemical problem involving blood sugar. More often then not, the glucose tolerance curve will look remarkably normal. Once again, variations in venous plasma pH over time will (in many cases far more than 4 to 7 hours) provide an important understanding of the underlying biochemical or metabolic disorder.

Ideally, four blood samples should be drawn over the course of 12 to 16 hours on the test day, and venous plasma pH should be determined at the time of each drawing. Furthermore, there is a specified meal plan which must be followed on the day of the test. Women who are cycling menstrually should undergo this type of venous plasma pH testing on three different days, where each day is representative of each phase within the menstrual cycle. The menstrual phase occurring between days 1 and 4; the pre-ovulatory phase occurring between days 5 and 14; and the premenstrual phase occurring between days 15 and 28. A more detailed description of venous plasma pH testing procedures and standardized food challenge tests is given in the "How To" section of this book in Chapter 9.

Dr. Atkins should be given credit for recognizing hypoglycemia as a problem which can result in "psychological" disturbances and in realizing that there may be various gradations of hypoglycemia. It is noteworthy that Dr. Atkins also suggests that his dietary therapy be revised to encompass a diet low in fat and relatively rich in complex carbohydrates in the event a patient responds poorly. In so suggesting, Dr. Atkins insightfully recognizes the possibility that hypoglycemia is not always the cause of a patient's distress.

In the case history below, the client makes mention of a book whose dietary guidelines she tried to follow. The title of that book is *Managing Your Mind and Mood Through Food* by Dr. Judith Wurtman. I will not attempt to review Dr. Wurtman's work here. It suffices to say that Dr. Wurtman offers recommendations which by and large are not completely inappropriate for alkaline types but are ineffective for acidic types.

LIFE HISTORY: BETWEEN TIME AND TIMBUKTU

Sharon was 41 years old and held a faculty position in physics at a local university. "I've been extremely run down and lately I've been missing my periods. I've also been suffering from a prolapsed mitral valve which gives me some severe arrhythmias and tachycardia. Sometimes I'll just lie awake at night. I can't sleep even though I'm exhausted when I go to bed. These problems seem to get worse premenstrually. I've never subscribed to psychological mumbo-jumbo, so when I read that a Ph.D. physicist was solving these problems using basic principles of physics and chemistry I decided to try BioBalancing.

I read Dr. Atkins book, *The Super Energy Diet* and it made a lot of sense. But the results I was getting were rather erratic. I'd feel well, then I'd feel worse. Reversing the high protein diet as his book suggested when I responded poorly seemed to help for awhile. Then I'd get sick again. At any rate I decided to stop fooling around with his concepts and pay a visit to a physician involved in treating hypoglycemia. He had me take a glucose tolerance test which showed that I was hypoglycemic. My blood sugar peaked in one hour and then dropped to levels below fasting one hour after that. I almost passed out during the test. To make a long story short the doctor put me on the high protein diet. Well, I got immediate results. Although I had to eat six small meals per day, I felt pretty well. My periods which at that time were 40 days apart at best, immediately became regular. That's when new problems began. My period started up like clockwork with only some minor cramping. When it started though I felt awful and continued feeling awful until ovulation. Remember all the problems I said I used to get during the premenstrual phase *before* I started the Atkins Diet?… migraines, nausea, the works. Well, after being on the Atkins Diet I'd get them *during* my menstrual and preovulatory phases. At ovulation it all cleared up and I felt well again… up until the time my period started up again. I thought it might have been an adjustment problem or a *healing crisis* (sound familiar?), but as I said, during my second cycle while on the Atkins Diet I once again felt great from day 15 through day 28 and then felt awful from day 1 through 14. I made another appointment to see my doctor. He said the hypo-glycemia was probably breaking through and that I should stay on my high protein diet no matter what. He also recommended that I take some supplements; inositol and vitamin E for my insomnia which was now developing from day 5 through 14. Good heavens, I almost died when I took them. The supplements made me feel far worse, to the point where I started to panic… that's just not me. I phoned the doctor, told him I was in bad shape and asked what I should do. He told me I had probably gone too far, said to discontinue the supplements and to reverse the diet, cut down on fat and protein and increase my carbohydrate intake. I tried that and felt much better… but only for a while. We tried a series of supplements, most of them did nothing and some of them, especially the inositol after my period made me feel worse.

So I quit the Atkins' scheme for a while and tried some of the tips that Judith Wurtman gives in her book, *Managing Your Mind and Mood through Food.* I figured with a Ph.D. and her affiliation with MIT (Massachusetts Institute of Technology) she ought to be a sharp cookie. What a let down! My PMS got so bad I damn near jumped out the window, and the reprieve I usually experience after my period starts wasn't as pronounced with Wurtman's dietary guidelines. And to think that she says that her guidelines are at best harmless! Anyway, that's about it. I've reached a dead end. I feel like there is no place for me. I'm suspended in limbo... nowhere. I thought maybe BioBalancing could help."

Sharon's metabolic profile proved to be quite interesting. She was extremely acidic from the day of ovulation (day 14-15) to the first day of menstruation (day 28-1). Thereafter, during the menstrual and preovulatory phases of her cycle (days 1 through 4 and 5 through 14 respectively) she was extremely alkaline. The Atkins Diet was therefore appropriate to some degree for Sharon's BioProfile only during one phase of her menstrual cycle, namely the premenstrual phase and at no other time. Sharon's doctor had mistakenly assumed that he had reversed Sharon's hypoglycemia. Sharon's switch from hypoglycemia (acidosis) to hyperglycemia (prediabetes or extreme alkalosis) was in fact *genetically programmed* and required a series of nutritional regimens, the application of each of which would coincide with the premenstrual, menstrual, and preovulatory phases of her cycle.

Sharon's results with BioBalancing were predictable. She remained on a nutritional regimen appropriate for acidic types during the premenstrual phase of her cycle, switching to a diet appropriate for alkaline types during the menstrual and preovulatory phases.

Three months of BioBalancing produced several benefits in addition to Sharon's renewed sense of well-being, and increased energy. She recovered from her insomnia and also lost 25 pounds.

This is how Sharon ate on a typical day when she was on the Super Energy Diet:

Breakfast: Poached egg, extra lean beef, 1 slice of diet bread, decaffeinated tea.

Snack: 1 hard boiled egg.

Lunch: Tuna salad with small amount of lettuce, thin slice of tomato, small amount of chopped onion, pepper and cucumber with oil and lemon dressing, weak tea.

Snack: Whole yogurt with dry roasted nuts.

Dinner: Chopped sirloin, peas and carrots with pat of butter, weak tea.

Snack: Diet bread with some peanut butter, small leftover portion of chopped sirloin.

You can see why this diet served to some extent to neutralize Sharon's acidity when she was premenstrual. From the examples I've already given you and from the information in the Appendix, you can see that while this diet is to some extent biased in favor acidic types, it does not go far enough in that it permits some inappropriate foods such as tomatoes, onions, peppers, cucumbers etc. Consequently, Sharon had to compensate for this error by relying on 6 small meals per day to keep her from drifting too far in the acid direction. *Acidic individuals who by definition are true hypoglycemics need only eat three meals a day to remain in BioBalance.*

The following describes Sharon's BioProfile when she adhered to the Super Energy Diet:

average menstrual pH (day 1 through 4) = 7.49

average preovulatory pH (day 5 through 14) = 7.50

average premenstrual pH (day 15 through 28) = 7.44

To some extent the Super Energy Diet stabilized Sharon's biochemistry during the premenstrual phase when she would otherwise have been excessively acidic, but it made her excessively alkaline during the menstrual and preovulatory phases.

When Sharon reversed her Super Energy Diet because of the distress she was encountering during the menstrual and preovulatory phases to a diet extremely rich in complex carbohydrates and almost devoid of meat, fish and poultry, her BioProfile looked like this:

average menstrual pH (day 1 through 4) = 7.45

average preovulatory pH (day 5 through 14) = 7.46

average premenstrual pH (day 15 through 28) = 7.40

This reversal stabilized Sharon's biochemistry during the menstrual and preovulatory phases when she would have otherwise been alkaline, but it made her excessively acidic during the premenstrual phase.

This is an example of how Sharon ate during a typical day while maintaining BioBalance during the premenstrual phase (day 15 through 28):

Breakfast: Chili with meat (very mildly seasoned), weak tea with cream.

Lunch: Salad containing, salmon and dark meat tuna, beans, artichoke hearts and carrots on a bed of spinach with olive oil, herbal tea.

Dinner: Spare ribs (very mildly seasoned), buttered brown rice, asparagus.

The supplements Sharon took during the premenstrual phase are listed in the Appendix in that section dealing with acidic biochemical types.

Clearly, Sharon did not need 6 meals per day during her premenstrual acid phase. The regimen outlined above is biased sufficiently in the alkaline inducing direction to have stabilized Sharon's biochemistry during the premenstrual phase. Her venous plasma pH during the premenstrual phase stabilized at 7.45 after Sharon engaged in BioBalance Therapy.

During both the menstrual phase (day 1 through 4) and the preovulatory phase (day 5 through 14) Sharon ate as follows while maintaining BioBalance:

Breakfast: Low fat yogurt (1%) with fresh citrus, regular coffee.

Lunch: Salad with low fat cottage cheese (1%), lettuce, onions, peppers, cucumbers and tomatoes, regular tea with lemon.

Dinner: Extra lean broiled pork chop, boiled potato with 1 pat of margarine (not butter), steamed broccoli.

The supplements Sharon took during her menstrual and preovulatory phases are listed in the Appendix in that section dealing with alkaline biochemical types.

Her venous plasma pH during her menstrual and preovulatory phases stabilized at 7.47.

CANDIDIASIS

Polysystemic chronic candidiasis also known as *candidiasis* is the medical terminology for a systemic yeast infection. Most physicians think that candidiasis or systemic yeast infections are strictly *female problems* resulting in vaginitis. Recent research has indicated that the narrow view taken by many physicians regarding candidiasis is far too restrictive. It has been my observation that candida albicans (yeast) does not discriminate between male and female, or young and old. Nor does it discriminate among various acid/alkaline biochemical types. The most common target for candida overgrowth is generally the reproductive tract in females and the gastrointestinal tract in both males and females. It is noteworthy that yeast commonly inhabits the human body and it is natural for yeast to do so. When I refer to a systemic yeast infection I am referring to a candida or a yeast overgrowth of the intestinal and genital tracts. Typically candida will ferment and transform simple carbohydrates or sugars and release chemical by-products into the human body and the human bloodstream. These by-products can have a noxious effect upon the central nervous system. It is not surprising that some Japanese researchers call candidiasis the *drunken man disorder*. It is not uncommon to hear many candida victims report that they continuously feel unpleasantly drowsy and generally impaired.

Dr. Orian Truss and Dr. William Crook are two advocates of the hypothesis that candida can in fact be responsible for many disorders whose symptoms generally appear to be of vague and nebulous origins tempting many physicians to diagnose these disorders as being of a psychological nature: depression, fatigue, anxiety, weight-related disorders, "feeling sick all over," etc. These physicians have recently captured the public's attention with the books, *The Yeast Connection* (Crook) and *The Missing Diagnosis* (Truss). The holistic health care community has recently followed suit and developed a check list/self-test where you can determine for yourself the odds of having candidiasis. The symptoms are multifaceted and can result in a profile similar to that of an individual who would be otherwise classified (and erroneously so) as having psychological problems.

The control of candidiasis varies depending upon the holistic physician with whom you consult. Typically candida control consists of a low carbohydrate diet or (and there is some controversy here) a diet whose moderate carbohydrate content consists only of complex carbohydrates so as to disrupt the yeast's life cycle. It is also suggested that the candidiasis victim ideally avoid yeast-bearing products (see asterisked items in the Appendix). In many cases a candicidal (candida-killing) medication is also administered in order to hasten the mortality of the candida infestation and overgrowth. Care must be given in using candicidals because in the process of killing off candida, antigenic material can be released into the bloodstream causing temporary nausea and disorientation. This phenomenon is known as the Herxheimer reaction in honor of the researcher who discovered it.

Because the candidiasis topic is currently quite hot and has attracted a good deal of public attention, people are naturally shocked when I say that the area of candida treatment has been overly emphasized. I often state that candida will be to the 1980s what hypoglycemia was to the 1970s. It was almost chic to state that your doctor had diagnosed you as hypoglycemic in the 1970s if you were generally feeling lousy. Today candidiasis is gaining favor. Candida treatment has in fact become so widespread within the holistic medical community that mainstream allopathic physicians refer to candidiasis as the "yuppie" disorder. Just about every other person who undergoes BioBalance Therapy initially claims that he or she has candidiasis.

Individuals are routinely screened for candida when undergoing BioBalance Therapy and, it is found that a significant number of these individuals are *asymptomatic* carriers. They carry high levels of candida, but have no symptoms at all *after* they are brought into BioBalance. Only a minority of individuals possess both a biochemical imbalance and candida overgrowth as well. The individual who possesses *both* candida overgrowth to which he or she is symptomatic and a biochemical imbalance, must sometimes be treated for both the candida overgrowth and the imbalance. I must however re-emphasize the fact that many individuals have been treated who possessed both a biochemical imbalance and candidiasis who responded very favorably to BioBalancing before any attempt was made to bring their candidiasis under control. This point is quite important, and I want to re-emphasize *that most individuals who have symptoms popularly associated with candidiasis do not have candidiasis but have instead a biochemical imbalance which lends itself to correction via BioBalancing.* This seems to indicate that in most cases (although certainly not all), BioBalancing is really all that is needed. Again, I cannot emphasize too strongly that polysystemic chronic candidiasis is a real disorder, but that its treatment has become abused to the point where most individuals being treated for candidiasis may be wasting their time and money.

I compare candidiasis with hypoglycemia in that hypoglycemia is also a real disorder. Recall, I mentioned earlier that extreme acidic types are hypoglycemic. But not *everyone* is extremely acidic, and many people with a biochemical imbalance may exhibit the symptoms of hypoglycemia. Hence claiming that *everyone* who exhibits vague, diffuse, undiagnosable symptoms is probably hypoglycemic is inaccurate. Similarly, stating that *everyone* who exhibits vague, diffuse, undiagnosable symptoms probably has polysystemic chronic candidiasis, is also inaccurate. *If of course you assume that individuals who have vague, diffuse, undiagnosable symptoms which have defied the medical profession probably have a biochemical imbalance of the acid/alkaline variety, then you will almost invariably be right.*

Physicians, especially holistic physicians are realizing that the candida cure is not everything it was cracked up to be initially. In fact, as the following case history demonstrates, some individuals get worse while "taking the cure." The Herxheimer reaction is often pointed to as the cause for a deteriorating condition. This is seldom the case. I contend the real cause consists of the physician's inadvertently giving the patient, whether he or she has candida or not, a diet *inappropriate* for his or her biochemical type.

Once again, I am respectful of the research currently being conducted regarding candidiasis. Incorporation of active candida control treatment as part of BioBalancing has raised the success rate of BioBalancing Therapy.

LIFE HISTORY: PLEASE PASS THE SUGAR

Andrea was 47 years old and 60 pounds overweight. She was also the mother of five. Aside from her pregnancies she could not recall when she last felt well.

"I'm living in a fog. Every day I just continuously push myself to get anything done and believe me with five children I just can't afford feeling this way. My husband's had it with me as well. I'm pretty sure he's seeing another woman." She stopped and began sobbing uncontrollably. When she recovered, she continued.

"In a way I can't blame him. The house is falling down around our ears, the kids are always on us. If I didn't feel so fantastic during my pregnancies, I would have had my tubes tied after our first child. I swear, I love the kids dearly, but they're so incredibly demanding. Sometimes I could wring their necks." She stopped and cried again. "My life is really a mess. I just feel absolutely horrible all the time. I guess dull or dim-witted is the best way to describe it. My body hurts and aches all over, really bad muscle pains, throbbing all the time. My chiropractor says I'm badly aligned. Who knows. My holistic doctor diagnosed candidiasis two years ago and I've been really good about my diet and my medication even though I overeat. I'm on Nystatin, you know? That's the medication my doctor says will kill the candida. I just don't get much better. I used to get rashes on my body, especially before my period, and sores — oh my God, just remembering them gives me the creeps. I still get them, but at least they're better. I still keep seeing my holistic doctor trying to get help. He changed my medication and put me on a new anticandida diet and told me to watch out for adverse reactions resulting from some kind of 'Herkimer' reaction or something, I think that was the word he used."

Andrea was politely told that the appropriate name for the adverse reaction to candicidals was the "Herxheimer" reaction. She was then asked about her diet.

"It's low in carbohydrates so the yeast won't be able to feed off the carbohydrates. I almost died. He said I should stick to it because the bad reaction was part of my discharge (sound familiar?) which he called that reaction I told you about. I did what he told me to do for two weeks. I mean I couldn't get out of bed. I just cried and cried all day. I told him I couldn't take it anymore. He said I had too much stress. So he sent me to a stress doctor who said I was acting out the role of a victim and martyr with my husband and even with the holistic doctor. He said that the doctor represents an authority figure. He said my problems probably relate back to my relationship with my father. He said I have a typical candida personality. I just can't believe it's true! Am I really that way? My dad loved me so much, he was such a caring man." She broke down again and cried again.

"I mean what am I supposed to do, the doctor says for me to go on the diet, try to make it through this Herkimer stuff, so I do. I try and now I'm some kind of nut for following directions. I know I'm not the brightest person in the world, but at least give me credit for trying."

Andrea was asked what happened when she went off the diet.

"That's the funny thing. I actually felt better. In fact, I just stopped eating because I just got tired of food completely. I fasted on and off for two weeks. I'm afraid to say it but I felt great and lost almost 20 pounds. I cleaned the house and actually enjoyed being with the kids. My husband was amazed. I know I still have sixty pounds to go. Hey, listen can't I just be fed through a tube or something so I can keep feeling the way I did when I fasted?"

Tests for candidiasis showed Andrea's levels to be quite elevated but more significantly they showed her to be extremely alkaline. Fasting incidentally is a very effective way to acidify your biochemistry. Alkaline types and some mixed types feel quite well and clear-headed when they fast. Fasting will generally, although not always, have the opposite effect on acidics. Through fasting, Andrea inadvertently locked onto a method of temporarily re-equilibrating her acid/alkaline biochemistry. It is also noteworthy that complex carbohydrates (and in a crisis situation even simple carbohydrates such as *sugar*) can acidify a person's biochemistry. Hence a low carbohydrate diet was the last thing in the world that Andrea needed. Her adverse reaction to her diet was *not* the Herxheimer reaction or any other type of discharge, but was an adverse reaction to her low carbohydrate intake. She had become so alkaline on her anti-candida diet that her central nervous system was being systematically deprived of oxygen.

Andrea called to cancel her next consultation at which she was to obtain her dietary recommendations. She was very agitated on the phone when she called and said that she felt "scary, depressed" and that she did not know if she could make it through the program. She was thinking of calling the local psychiatric center for emergency treatment. She was asked what she had eaten that morning.

"Last night we went out and I had steak and lobster tails with cream of cauliflower soup and drawn butter. This morning I had leftovers. I can't take this anymore! Maybe it's *just me!*" She broke down and cried uncontrollably on the phone.

If you check the Appendix you'll see that this type of food is absolutely contraindicated for someone as alkaline as Andrea. Despite her candidiasis, her crisis called for emergency intervention, but not of a psychiatric variety. She was asked to drink a large glass of regular coffee with *three heaping teaspoons of sugar.*

Her response was one of surprise. "Huh? I mean won't that sugar make my candida go crazy." She was told that it might in the long run, but the immediate objective consisted of lessening her severe alkaline imbalance. She did as she was instructed, called back fifteen minutes later and said she felt better even though she was still far from feeling 100%. She did feel well enough to keep her appointment. She was advised to fast for as long as she felt comfortable before starting on her nutritional regimen.

The results were predictable. She fasted for almost two weeks and reported feeling "terrific." After the termination of her program six months later, Andrea was very different from the person who initially sought assistance.

"I feel great! I've lost 60 pounds and my skin has cleared up. Do I ever have energy! I'm taking up day care to earn some money and because I realize that I really love kids and that's what I want to do with my life. I also joined a Bible study group in the evenings. My husband doesn't like that too much, but that's the way it goes. I forgive him for how he acted, but there's just too much I want to do with my life and I simply can't afford to sit around any longer and feel depressed and sorry for myself."

Andrea's BioProfile while she was undergoing treatment for her candidiasis was characterized by an average venous plasma pH of 7.52 irrespective of her cycle phase.

This is an example of how Andrea ate on a typical day while she was undergoing treatment for her candidiasis:

Breakfast: All natural wheat free/yeast free cereal with nuts and mashed tofu, distilled water.

Lunch: Fresh salmon, steamed corn (fresh) and potato, distilled water.

Dinner: Beef, lentils, broccoli, unleavened bread (Essene bread), mineral water.

Andrea's BioProfile after she achieved BioBalance was characterized by an average venous plasma pH of 7.45 irrespective of her cycle phase.

This is an example of how Andrea ate on a typical day during and after she achieved BioBalance:

Breakfast: Fresh citrus fruit, regular coffee with 1 teaspoon of sugar.

Lunch: Garden salad with lettuce, shredded cabbage, tomatoes, onions, cucumbers, peppers, raw broccoli, small amount of safflower oil (no salt), fresh squeezed lemon, sprinkling of vinegar, regular coffee with 1 teaspoon of sugar.

Dinner: Low fat yogurt, fresh fruit, garden salad (see lunch above), steamed broccoli, onions and brown rice, herbal tea.

Andrea took supplements appropriate for alkaline types as described in the Appendix. Because Andrea was very alkaline her regimen rarely included any meat, fish or poultry. Her source of protein was largely low fat and skim dairy. Accordingly she added 10 micrograms of B12 to her supplements to avoid incurring a B12 deficiency in the long term. In looking at the Appendix, you will note that doses of supplemental vitamin B12 substantially higher than 10 micrograms would not otherwise be appropriate for alkaline types such as Andrea.

THE FEINGOLD DIET

The Feingold Diet has become something of a sacred cow and therefore to attack it will likely only result in wrath from some members of the public.

However, I am not attacking the Feingold Diet. In a nutshell Dr. Feingold has observed that the behavior of hyperkinetic-learning disabled (H-LD) children improves significantly if they stop eating foods with artificial colorings, flavorings and additives. I cannot state too emphatically that I am *not* a spokesman for artificial additives, flavorings and colorings. In the ideal world we would rid our foods of all questionable substances in the same fashion that Drs. Ringsdorf and Cheraskin advocate that we rid ourselves of all junk food. Unfortunately we do not live in the ideal world and completely eliminating additives of this nature from an H-LD child's diet can be exasperating. Having an H-LD child can be exasperating enough. I am also not denying Dr. Feingold's observations. Based upon the impact of BioBalance Therapy on H-LD children, I would guess that if a child is hyperkinetic-learning disabled he is not likely to be in BioBalance and therefore he is also likely to suffer severe behavioral reactions to additives which other individuals may tolerate reasonably well in small doses. It has been my observation that when hyperkinetic learning disabled children are brought into BioBalance they become far more tolerant of those agents that Dr. Feingold proposes be eliminated from the diet. The question parents are faced with is perhaps not whether BioBalancing or the Feingold Diet is in fact correct or best, but rather *which of the two strategies is easier to implement and more effective.* As it is with the case of food allergies, so it is also probably the case with additives. BioBalance tends to reduce sensitivities to foods which will otherwise result in behavioral problems. These problems are of course almost invariably misdiagnosed as being psychological in origin.

Life History: Will the Real Adam Please Step Forward

Adam was 11 years old and hyperactive. Hyperactive may be too weak a word to use. Adam gave new meaning to the word hyperactivity. His mother, Linda was visibly distraught as Adam rapidly examined everything in the consultation room while he hummed and talked to himself at a frenetic pace. At one point, Adam's father had to escort him out after he knocked over a large plant and began kicking at the walls.

Linda was practically in tears. "It's been this way ever since I can remember. Only now it's getting worse as he gets closer to puberty. He's been on and off of medication. I just don't like the idea of medicating a child Adam's age. My husband and I have been at our wits' end. His behavior has had a poor effect upon his brother and sister who are not hyperactive, incidentally. Adam is very trying. I can't tell you how much money we've spent on physicians, psychiatrists and specialists. It's been awful. I majored in psychology in college, so naturally I thought his problem might be psychological. We went to see a number of psychiatrists and psychologists specializing in children's problems and family therapy. Adam's the middle child so the middle child syndrome hypothesis seemed to make sense. I don't know, it makes sense on paper I guess but *no amount of psychotherapy seems to help.*"

"Then we heard about the Feingold Diet so we tried that. It actually helped a bit at first, but then Adam fell right back into the same rut. Let me tell you, you just don't know how many additives, preservatives and how much junk there is in food until you're made aware of it. He's still on the Feingold Diet, for insurance's sake. I suppose it's a good idea for him not to eat junk. But it's so hard especially since he gets into everything at school. He goes to a special school by the way. The school's nutritionist had the cafeteria make special arrangements for Adam. We also looked at food allergies, but the idea of rotating foods, restricting his diet further and eliminating junk foods to boot all at once is absolutely mind boggling. Sometimes I think we just *did something wrong*. But I just don't know what. Maybe *it's just Adam*, I mean maybe *it's just him*. When will he *learn to take responsibility* for his actions. Anyway my husband and I heard that the BioBalance Diet is not as tough. You know, no specialty foods or anything so that I don't have to become a slave to my kitchen. So I figured that we'd try the Dr. Wiley/BioBalance Diet out."

Linda was told that while some health care professionals advocate "THE DIET," there is no such thing as The BioBalance Diet, but that each diet must be tailored to fit an individual's BioProfile. It appeared she understood. You will see shortly that she did not.

Adam's biochemical profile spelled big trouble. His acid/alkaline biochemical imbalance oscillated over a 24 hour period. He was extremely alkaline in the morning and extremely acidic in the evening. I say this is trouble because administering BioBalance nutritional therapy to children is difficult enough. Children most often gravitate toward foods they like to eat and not foods which are necessarily biochemically appropriate or "good" for them regardless of what they are told. Having two children of my own (who are not hyperkinetic) I know exactly how tough it is. While adults may state that they'll eat dirt if that's what it takes to get well, children don't operate that way. Adam's case was going to be particularly tough because in effect there were three Adams, the early morning extremely alkaline Adam, the transient midafternoon mixed type Adam, and the evening extremely acidic Adam.

It was suggested that Linda try feeding Adam a diet appropriate for each type during each respective portion of the day. It was pointed out that Adam's dietary regimens were not as complex as they appeared in that Adam had the widest variety of foods to choose from in the midafternoon when he was at school. Linda was also told that while additives and preservatives are best excluded, they had sadly become a fact of life and only a strong grass roots political/economic movement could curb their use. Accordingly, it was suggested that Linda ease up on some of the Feingold restrictions after she noted an improvement in Adam's behavior. Follow up consultations showed that Adam had improved substantially indeed. His grades had gone up from a C average to a B+ over a two semester period. This was the first time such an improvement had ever occurred. His teachers and his school psychologist, all unaware of the fact that he was involved in a program of BioBalancing, had commented on his improved behavior. Linda was very pleased. "Adam is doing so well. There are times he relapses a bit, but it's always when he starts eating the wrong foods especially later in the day." Like some enlightened teachers, Linda had learned to observe the relationship between what children ate and their behavior and academic performance.

It is noteworthy that because Adam started his downward acid/ alkaline slide into extreme acidosis in the later afternoon, those foods which were most inimical to him at that time were foods commonly found in school vending machines such as candy bars and even "wholesome" foods like fruits, foods which he could tolerate with greater impunity in the morning, and not at all by late afternoon. Nonetheless, with the exception of fruits, these foods have no nutritive value and I wouldn't recommend them for anyone.

Linda went on. "Some friends of mine whose children are also hyperkinetic will be trying BioBalancing out with their kids too. My friend Sylvia is especially interested in BioBalancing. The problem is, she placed her little boy Michael on Adam's diet and he actually got worse! I don't understand this. I thought that this diet was appropriate for hyperactive children. Why should Michael get worse? Do you suppose Michael's problems *really are* psychological?" As you can see, although Linda was ready to embrace BioBalance Therapy for Adam she still missed the point that Adam's diet could not be generalized to every hyperkenetic child.

The following describes Adam's BioProfile when he was adhering to the Feingold Diet:

early morning pH	= 7.52
mid morning pH	= 7.49
mid day pH	= 7.44
mid afternoon pH	= 7.42
evening pH	= 7.39

It suffices to say that Adam's regimen while on the Feingold diet was as additive free and preservative free as is possible.

Adam's BioProfile after he achieved BioBalance was characterized by a constant pH in the immediate neighborhood of 7.44. This is an example of how Adam ate on a typical day both during BioBalance Therapy and after he achieved BioBalance; (recall BioBalance Therapy is not curative, but is instead a method of controlling underlying acid/alkaline imbalances):

> Breakfast: Whole grain bread, fresh squeezed citrus juice and regular coffee with skim milk, 1 teaspoon of sugar.
>
> Lunch: Peanut butter on diet sliced whole grain bread, Jarlsberg cheese, cup of home made beef stock, whole milk.
>
> Afternoon Snack: Cheese and dry roasted nuts, cashew butter on an apple slice.
>
> Dinner: Chopped sirloin, home made baked beans with bacon, buttered baked potato, *dilute* apple juice.

Adam took supplements appropriate for alkaline types in the morning, supplements appropriate for mixed types in the afternoon and supplements for acidic types in the evening. See the Appendix.

EAT TO WIN

Sports medicine has rapidly become Big Business. Sports nutrition is gradually becoming Big Business too. Among all the sports nutrition books, Dr. Robert Haas's book, *Eat to Win (The Sports Nutrition Bible)* stands out. Dr. Haas's book probably became a best seller in part because his program is endorsed by Martina Navratilova, the international tennis champion. As it turns out, Dr. Haas's program probably helped save Martina's life and likely went very far to improve her tennis game. You shouldn't be terribly surprised when I state in the same breath that I know that the *Eat to Win* approach can make you feel as though you're half dead and mess up your tennis game as well if it happens to be inappropriate for your BioProfile.

Instead of discussing *Eat to Win* in any detail, let's see if you can determine the acid/alkaline subgroup which would benefit from it, given a summary description of the diet that put Martina over the top. Martina claims that she's eating "piles of pasta, potatoes, rice and bread." Any clues? Dr. Haas also seems to imply that if his approach works for some people, it must work for everyone. After all, the Haas program worked for Jimmy Connors, Fred Stolle, Gene Mayer, Nancy Lieberman and the James and Jonathan DiDonnato twins... it's got to work for you... right? Having come this far, the shortcomings of the Haas program should be evident to you.

Dr. Haas individualizes his program by making it person-specific. This specificity does not however take acid/alkaline biochemistry into account. If you recall what I've repeatedly said in this book you will understand what I'm about to say. *Martina Navratilova simply lucked out by adhering to the Haas program.*

LIFE HISTORY: BREAKFAST OF CHAMPIONS

Norm was 29 years old and a real loser. A loser at jogging... a loser at tennis... a loser at golf... and more recently, a big loser on the corporate battlefield. Norm read all the *right* books on nutrition and health, including *Eat to Win* and *Eat to Succeed* but the nutritional approaches advocated by these books seemed to make him feel worse. Norm couldn't figure out why a program that helped superstars couldn't do anything for him but make him feel awful. He had been to half a dozen "sports psychiatrists" who had him believing that he couldn't succeed because he didn't want to succeed. Norm was too smart to buy into that for very long so he decided to try BioBalancing.

"I used to be a real superstar when I was a kid. I was good at any sport I went out for. But now, I'm wasted. I don't think I could score at hop scotch. Hell, I can't even score in bed with my girlfriend. It used to be that we had a running joke. Wanna know the difference between a young man, a middle aged man and an old man? The young man will do it triweekly. The middle aged guy will try weekly, and the old guy will just try weakly. I don't think they invented a category for me. I feel like a fossil. I don't get it. I do all the *right stuff* and all I get is the shaft. I really feel like hell. How I even manage to get on the tennis courts or go to work in the morning is a total mystery to me."

It was a mystery to me too. His venous plasma pH averaged 7.39 which is extremely acidic. It was surprising that Norm wasn't hallucinating in a mental care facility. Norm did things by the book. In this case his book was "The Sports Nutrition Bible," namely *Eat to Win* and the book *Eat to*

Succeed. He had stuck to the guidelines in these books for over a year. Sure enough, Norm's eating patterns mimicked those in both books and sure enough, Norm was getting increasingly acidic and feeling worse by the week.

Unlike many other individuals who are acidic, Norm's reaction to his BioBalance guidelines was one of enthusiasm. Norm was a pragmatist. If it worked, he'd go with it. If it failed, he'd drop it. Norm was cracking up with laughter, none of it sarcastic.

"O.K.! That's what I call great eating. Liver, bacon and eggs for breakfast. Breakfast of champions! Steak and beans for lunch, sausage and veggies for dinner… all right! Right on! Wait 'till they hear about this at the health club… there gonna think that BioBalancing is for quackos and whackos! See if I give a damn, as long as I feel better."

Better wasn't the word for it. It took a little more than six weeks for Norm to shape up. His venous plasma pH stabilized at 7.47. He did beautifully. He was only too happy to admit to his victories.

"Frigging A all the way! I'm unbeatable at tennis and golf. They can't stop me at marathons. I've even signed up for the Iron Man competition… oh and by the way, it's tri *daily* now!." Norm couldn't sit still; he was clearly elated and exuberant. "My buddies at the club and at the office told me I'd drop dead of a stroke if I kept up with this BioBalance stuff. I told them I wouldn't, but frankly who gives a damn. I fired all of my shrinks. I'm feeling great!"

It would be of little value to continue with lengthy case histories of individuals' experiences with other currently popular forms of dietary therapy. What follows are instead brief descriptions of several dietary therapies given within the context of BioBalancing. I leave it to you to test yourself and determine for which biochemical type each dietary therapy is best suited. To check yourself you may wish to review the "Consumer's Guide to Nutritional Therapy" as listed in Chapter 4.

PSYCHODIETETICS/ORTHOMOLECULAR MEDICINE

The underlying assumption advanced by Drs. Cheraskin and Ringsdorf in the book *Psychodietetics*, consists of the fact that diet is primarily responsible for problems commonly classified as "psychological." The authors espouse an approach popularized by a branch of medicine called orthomolecular medicine (loosely translated meaning, making the molecules fit correctly).

Specifically, the authors advocate placing the patient on what they call THE OPTIMAL DIET and generally giving the patient vitamin-mineral supplements along with dietary advice. The sources which the authors cite are impressive. Furthermore, THE OPTIMAL DIET would likely seem reasonable, rational and well balanced to most nutritionists and physicians. Yet again, the term "well balanced" is completely relative and should be gauged to your BioProfile.

THE OPTIMAL DIET as loosely defined in the book *Psychodietetics* is one which is devoid of junk food or foods low in nutritional value and generally loaded with unnecessary chemical additives. The authors of *Psychodietetics* are more sophisticated than this of course, but still they do not include the subtle yet profound impact of deviations in biochemical type which are part and parcel of BioBalancing's classification scheme. According to the *Psychodietetics* guidelines, coffee, grapefruit, dairy and baked filet of sole would be among some foods found to be acceptable.

Perhaps the biggest contribution made by *Psychodietetics* consists of raising public awareness to the problems of chronic consumption of junk food and processed food. This contribution is especially noteworthy in that at the time Cheraskin and Ringsdorf wrote this book most people believed that food had little if any effect on our state of well-being. This belief was at that time also shared by the medical community. In essence these authors were pioneers espousing a viewpoint either unsupported by conventional wisdom or attacked by special interest groups.

THE DR. BERGER IMMUNE POWER DIET/THE DR. RANDOLPH ALLERGEN FREE ELIMINATION-ROTATION DIET

The idea that psychological problems could be the result of allergies has been put into widespread practice by Dr. Theron Randolph. Oftentimes individuals think of allergies as resulting in runny noses, sneezing, wheezing and itchy eyes. Dr. Randolph has found that allergies may oftentimes be caused by foods as well as by environmentally borne substances that can result in more insidious malfunctions manifesting themselves as problems, commonly referred to as 'behavioral' or 'psychological.' Dr. Randolph typically fasts an individual in a hypoallergenic environment and then reintroduces foods in isolated and sequential order to see how a patient reacts. Dr. Randolph and others also believe that an individual can become allergic to a food if it or a member of the food family to which that food belongs is eaten too frequently or repeatedly. Consequently, Dr. Randolph advocates an allergen elimination/ rotation strategy whereby suspected allergens are eliminated, then reintroduced to confirm their offending status and finally (if possible) eaten only infrequently and rotated in time with other foods so as to eliminate or minimize deleterious effects.

Dr. Stuart Berger has taken aspects of Dr. Randolph's approach a step further and has, in a sense, attempted to derive a generalized format and diet/program which anyone can use in order to identify potential allergens. He also advocates supplementation with vitamins, minerals and amino acids "to boost one's immune system," whereas Dr. Randolph seems to tacitly argue against the introduction of supplements because they may contain allergic substances, such as fillers, colors, binders, etc. The types of vitamins, minerals and amino acids one takes depend upon one's score on an "IQ test" ("immune quotient test"), which gauges how you feel and what your eating habits are. It also uses one's sex, age and a list of other factors, *none of which pertain to acid/alkaline biochemistry*. Adverse reactions, Dr. Berger believes are the result of *detoxification* which will yield substantial benefits if successfully weathered. All in all, Dr. Berger believes that a combination allergen elimination/rotation diet in conjunction with supplementation is the key to increased well-being and a fortified immune system. Typically, Dr. Berger's guidelines consist of diets which are carbohydrate rich and which are supplemented with a full spectrum vitamin/mineral supplement which is especially biased in favor of the B vitamins (especially B1, B2 and B6).

WEIGHT MAINTENANCE

BioBalancing is absolutely critical if you wish to embark on a successful program of weight maintenance. Most weight maintenance diets don't work because they do not address an individual's fundamental need which consists of achieving BioBalance. Most people who lose weight simply put it right back on. That's precisely why weight loss and diet centers gross fortunes every year.

Reducing caloric intake and eating "sensibly" or eating "wonderful" and "wholesome" foods is no guarantee of anything. Worse yet, as I've already shown you, eating 'light' to lose weight can be catastrophic if you are not alkaline. Weight maintenance involves stabilization of your weight at or around that weight at which you feel most comfortable. Most of the individuals with weight problems who engage in a program of BioBalancing are obese. Typically, the obese person will have been failed by virtually every imaginable diet, fad and craze. He or she (usually she) will feel guilty and will be told by friends and relatives that she is lacking "will power."

I like to tell audiences when I'm invited to speak, that in the context of BioBalancing and weight control, the last time I saw Will Power, he was sneaking out the back door at a weight loss clinic. Guilt and frustration mark the life of the obese person. I will not relate another case history here. Andrea's case history discussed earlier could be viewed as a case history regarding obesity. It is fair to say that the majority of women who get involved with BioBalancing are overweight. While Andrea was only 60 pounds overweight when she first started her program, BioBalancing has worked with individuals who have been more than 100 pounds overweight. To the uninitiated, when BioBalance is achieved, weight loss becomes "magically" and "mysteriously" simple and requires some planning but little if any will power.

The first thought that comes to mind where weight loss is concerned is that somehow individuals who undergo BioBalance Therapy to lose weight will lose it more effortlessly because somehow they are using *power of suggestion*. Power of suggestion in this context is also known as the *placebo* effect. If you read my research published in the *International Journal of Biosocial Research* (see references) you will see that power of suggestion has been experimentally tested in BioBalance Therapy and plays little if any role.

The moral of this story is pretty straightforward. If you want to engage in a successful weight management program, you should engage in a program of BioBalancing.

THE PREMENSTRUAL SYNDROME (PMS) DIET

By this time you should realize that there is no such thing as The PMS Diet, because it is rare to find two women who have PMS and are biochemically identical. Nonetheless, the popular press and some branches of the medical community are still searching for the nutritional Holy Grail by looking for *The* PMS Diet.

Women comprise more than 70% of those seeking assistance through BioBalancing. This is not an accident since biochemical imbalance is genetic and female sex-linked imbalances seem to express themselves more decisively than their male counterparts. Hence, a woman's hormonal configuration will accentuate or amplify an underlying set of biochemical imbalances. This generally does not pose a problem insofar as BioBalance Therapy is concerned since there exists a nutritional countermeasure for every type of acid/alkaline imbalance regardless of its severity.

I am not being derisive nor am I stereotyping when I say that *on the average*, women who are not BioBalanced are more diseased than their male counterparts. I believe the statistics will bear me out. The severity of biochemical imbalance usually varies in accordance with a woman's menstrual cycle. It would be impossible and counterproductive to tell you all of the diets previously tried by the women who have gone through BioBalance Therapy for the treatment of PMS. One diet does however stand out, namely the diet advocated by Dr. Ronald Norris, M.D. in his book *PMS, Premenstrual Syndrome*. Dr. Norris's nutritional recommendations are really guidelines more than an actual diet. They are broad enough to have some therapeutic value. These guidelines include reduction of fat intake and elimination of some foods such as: smoked fish (typically, herring, sardines and salmon), fatty meats, artichokes and some legumes. These guidelines also include increased intake of the vitamins B1, B2 and B6 which are implied to be the anti-PMS vitamins or the *energy* vitamins.

In discussing PMS in general, Dr. Norris points out that women should be prescreened for PMS as well as for a host of other problems that might be psychological in nature. This position may result from the fact that Dr. Norris is a psychiatrist by training. Accordingly, he has each patient take a battery of psychological tests which are analyzed by a psychologist to determine if a patient may require counseling for a psychological problem as well. I will show you later why I disagree with this approach.

In the context of BioBalancing it is safe to say that while PMS in severe forms may shatter social relationships and result in *secondary* stress, stress is rarely a cause or a contributory factor in PMS. This statement may seem counter-intuitive to you. It is nonetheless correct as I will demonstrate to you later. Briefly, it is found that women who are not in BioBalance are likely to have PMS or some other type of "emotional" disorder remarkably similar to PMS. These emotional disorders can be aggravated by social stress. This statement incidentally is not in contradiction with the remark I just made, because women who are brought into BioBalance reach their peak performance potential, are generally free of disabling emotional disorders and have a much higher tolerance to stress.

ONE WHO KEPT THE FAITH

My undergraduate college history professor used to tell me that if I wanted to start an argument and create enemies all I had to do was discuss religion or politics. I attended undergraduate school in the mid and late '60's. Today a discussion of nutrition can alone create as much tension and hostility as a discussion of *both* religion and politics.

The Pritikin Program has gained substantial popularity. I have met more than a few devotees of Pritikin's philosophy who would likely defend their beliefs to the death. While I emphasize (yet again) that the Pritikin program does benefit some individuals (alkaline types), it can deleteriously affect others (mixed and acidic types). I have seen some mixed and acidic acquaintances zealously embrace a Pritikin lifestyle and psychologically erode. Nonetheless they are prepared to wage a holy war against anyone who might insinuate that the Pritikin program is limited in its efficacy and can in fact be disastrous if inappropriately applied. A friend of mine in particular has become increasingly hyper and nervous since becoming a Pritikin convert. He can hardly sleep and he is bickering with increased frequency with his wife as well as with his business associates and friends. He claims this "electric energy" is part of his "new found assertive self." I know better and can testify to the fact that he is bionutritionally running himself into the ground and courting a nervous breakdown. Yet everytime the discussion comes around to nutrition he excitedly points to his flat, rock hard belly and tells me he'll outlive all of BioBalancing's clients. Perhaps he will and perhaps he won't. In either event his longevity (or lack of it) will prove little if anything.

My friend's case is not singular. I have thus far discussed a number of case histories. The following case history recounts the story of a noble but failed attempt to escape the paralyzing grip of nutritional dogma. It describes an individual who could not make a break with popular, conventional and *self-evident* nutritional wisdom. As you will see, while there is an element of humor in this case, it is tragic in the final analysis.

Phoebe was a 52 year old certified nutritionist. She had been suffering from panic attacks for more than 30 years. Phoebe related a rather fascinating story.

"I checked out some credentials here. I called various institutions and I found out that the people behind BioBalancing aren't certified nutritionists. My contact suggested that I not waste my time and money with BioBalancing. She said it was just another quack fad. She said that I should seek out assistance from a certified dietician... *a real expert.* Nevertheless I have an open mind and I decided to give this BioBalance thing a shot. I'll tell my friends that BioBalancing's my 'snake oil', no offense intended." She continued by describing her problem.

"I've always been a nervous person. But in my late 20's I had my first panic attack. My life hasn't been the same since. I've seen dozens of physicians. I think they all went to the same school of medicine; each of them told me I was *within normal limits*. That's become a joke to me. Then I went through just about every form of psychotherapy you can imagine. You might say I was psychotherapy-crazy. I even consulted with a real Viennese Freudian analyst. The whole schtick... beard, pipe, accent, couch... very charming old world style. Nothing helped."

Phoebe went on. "See these shoes?," she said, pointing to her track shoes. I've seen some very exotic track shoes in recent years but Phoebe's took first prize. They had far more rubber grip than they had suede uppers. At a glance the soles seemed to put the tread on a farm tractor to shame. Phoebe discussed her rationale for these unusual shoes. "I don't jog but I like to know my feet are planted firmly on the ground. I got these shoes at a specialty outlet. You see, sometimes I get so panicky that I feel as though I'm going to fly off into outer space or some other dimension so I get comfort out of being well grounded. Please don't laugh." Phoebe was clearly in distress. "I've always been panicky," she said, "but as of three years ago it's gotten worse. So bad in fact I've started taking antipsychotic medication. It seems to be situation-specific. I get panicky if I feel trapped either in a closed space or in a situation I can't get out of." She was asked to be more specific about her problem. The information she supplied was revealing.

"Well, let's see. Three years ago I decided I was going to start *eating right*, you know follow a lot of the sensible guidelines, cut way back on red meat, reduce my fat intake, concentrate more on unsaturated fats, eat more grains and fresh fruits and vegetables."

She was asked to describe a typical day insofar as her eating habits were concerned. "Well, breakfast is usually a whole grain cereal with some fruit and low fat milk, usually 1% milk or skim and a grain beverage. Caffeine's bad for you, you know... oh, and a slice of whole grain bread fresh baked at the natural food bakery. Fiber's important. O.K. Let's see, lunch is usually a tossed salad, a hard boiled egg or some lean poultry or fish and sometimes some cheese, but not too much. I want to make sure my fat intake isn't too high. That brings us to dinner, some light fish or chicken breast, a baked potato or whole grain, and a vegetable. You've got to admit I eat pretty well."

It wasn't clear that Phoebe was eating "well" at all. Perhaps Phoebe's definition of wellness conformed to that definition endorsed by the "real experts" but it did not conform to any definition of wellness within the context of BioBalancing. Phoebe was eating foods appropriate for alkaline biochemical types. Given the fact that she was suffering significant psychological disease, it was immediately apparent that she was decidedly *not* alkaline but was either a mixed type and driven to an acidic state by her diet, or (even worse) she was acidic and driven to an extreme acidic state by her diet. In either event, the only non-nutritive way Phoebe could possibly weather the biochemical storm to which she was nutritionally subjecting herself was by taking antipsychotic medication. Absent that medication, Phoebe might very well mentally fly off into orbit irrespective of the heavy duty traction on her shoes.

Subsequent analyses indicated that with an average venous plasma pH of 7.41, Phoebe was both extremely acidic and subsequent analyses also indicated that she had a severe case of candidiasis as well. When she was given her nutritional recommendations she was predictably stunned. "I'm really disappointed. I thought maybe I'd be told to stop eating a few foods I'm now eating like navy beans or something. But this! I mean this diet has cholesterol with a capital C. I'm being told to eat just the *opposite* of what I've been accustomed to. I'm very skeptical."

Twenty/twenty hindsight, otherwise known as Monday morning quarterbacking, is a marvelous thing. If Phoebe had given BioBalance Therapy a chance, she might have been told to read *Dr. Atkins' Super Energy Diet* in that the Atkins diet is not totally dissimilar to the diet outlined for Phoebe, and because it is advocated by a "real" doctor, skeptics sometimes feel reassured.

Phoebe deliberated long and hard in deciding whether to follow through. Amusingly and sadly, shortly after Phoebe's consultation the following episode unfolded at the local health food store which Phoebe frequented. Phoebe stopped by and asked the owner about BioBalancing while making a purchase. "Do you know anything about this BioBalance stuff? I mean is it on the level or is it some kind of quack scam? I just can't believe intelligent people would suggest that I start eating red meat." The store owner immediately jumped to BioBalancing's defense. "All I can tell you is that most people I know who go through with BioBalancing feel about 100% better regardless of the fact that its methods seem unconventional."

Poor Phoebe got it from both barrels. As it turned out, Megan, a young successful businesswoman and one of BioBalancing's former clients was also present and overheard this conversation. Megan enthusiastically spoke up, "Hey, I've been through BioBalance Therapy and I feel great. I eat red meat almost every day. Before I changed my diet I was nervous, run down and headaches were part of my life. It's not quackery!"

Phoebe was perplexed. But what was BioBalancing in contrast with recommendations made by *real* and *accredited experts*? In Phoebe's mind BioBalancing was formulated by a bunch of lunatics. To conclude my story, Phoebe cancelled her next appointment. Her parting words were polite, "I'm sure BioBalancing works for some people; it's just not for me."

The moral of this story consists of the fact that conventional wisdom presented as *intuitively obvious* by the *experts* dies hard. As far as can be determined, Phoebe virtuously persists in her dietary habits, pops antipsychotic medication and wears her elaborate Flash Gordon-type track shoes that grip life's highway and keep her from mentally blasting off into the twilight zone.

Historically, Isaac Newton built upon Galileo's laws to revolutionize physics. Newton's physics was immediately accepted not primarily because of its elegance in mathematically describing the earth's motion around the sun but because it was *practical* and proved very useful to the British army and navy in plotting artillery trajectories when engaging the enemy. Long after Newton's methods became well established, the philosopher *experts* of Newton's day were still pontificating and bickering among themselves regarding the merits of Newtonian science. These arguments are now at best anecdotal. History has long forgotten them. While my own insights pale substantially when compared with Galileo's and Newton's, I suspect that the future of nutrition and medicine will unfold in similar fashion... persecuted heretics... proven theories producing practical, *cost effective* results... accredited *experts* becoming intellectual casualties in the wake of revolution. You see, one way or another, history always repeats itself. As President Harry Truman said, the only thing that's new is the history you don't know!

V

BioBalance and Cyclic Disorders

At a lecture I gave on BioBalancing much of the information provided in Chapters 1 and 2 was discussed with the audience. Understandably, I was somewhat frustrated and taken aback when a woman in the audience asked me after my lecture, "Okay, what do I eat?" She was visibly perplexed when I told her that I hadn't the vaguest idea. Her spouse seemed to understand as little of my lecture as she did when he stated, "There's the Dr. Feingold Diet, the Pritikin Diet, the Dr. Berger Diet... so what's the Dr. Wiley Diet?" I insisted that there was no such thing as the Dr. Wiley Diet or the BioBalance Diet, for that matter. They both looked puzzled but still wouldn't give up. She then proceeded to describe her symptoms. While I always try to be polite and conceal my frustration, I'm sure it makes itself apparent when people demand that I conduct instantaneous diagnoses. I told her that symptoms alone were insufficient in enabling me to make a diagnosis because as I had already pointed out in my lecture it is possible for two individuals to possess identical symptoms and yet possess different types and degrees of biochemical imbalance. I reiterated the fact that individuals have uniquely different fingerprints, uniquely different signatures, and may have uniquely different biochemical profiles. I pointed to the fact that while both Ann and Melissa, (whose cases I have discussed in Chapter 2) suffered from attacks of panic, they were biochemically very different people whose nutritional regimens as formulated in their respective programs of BioBalance Therapy were radically different as well.

Conversely, I also pointed out that sometimes two individuals might exhibit different symptoms and yet possess remarkably similar biochemical profiles and could thus be treated in similar fashion through the use of BioBalancing. These points only seemed to mystify this couple and they walked away somewhat baffled and disappointed in my not having given them *THE* DIET.

A simpler way of explaining the fact that BioBalancing does not provide *THE* DIET is through the analogy that *one size does not fit all* or that "one man's meat is another man's poison." This concept is readily understood until the plot thickens when I state that sometimes one size does not even fit the same person day after day. Similarly, one man's (or woman's) meat on a certain day may well turn out to be that same man's (or woman's) poison on another day.

If you have understood the foundations of BioBalancing which I have outlined for you in Chapters 1 and 2, you might then ask "Okay, what am I, acid or alkaline?" But you will recall that there are individuals (such as Maria) whose acid/alkaline biochemistry *shifts gears* either from one extreme to another or from a moderate to a severe imbalance at different times of the day, month or year. As you are about to see, this problem while predominant among women on a monthly basis, is not peculiar to women who suffer from premenstrual syndrome more commonly known as PMS. In order to understand the significance of cyclic disorders it is critical for you to understand that it is possible for an individual's acid/alkaline imbalance to change despite the fact that his or her nutritional regimen may *not* have appreciably changed. The underlying cause for this *shift in biochemical gears* is genetic. The psychophysiological "disease" resulting from genetic causes, is enhanced in turn as a result of *inappropriate* nutrition. Note that I did not say *poor* nutrition or malnutrition, but rather nutrition *inappropriate for your biochemical type.* Hence if you are afflicted with a cyclic disorder you will by definition respond well to one nutritional regimen for a certain period of time and then respond poorly to that same regimen for another period of time.

Maria, whose case history was briefly mentioned in Chapter 2 was such an individual. Favorable response to one nutritional regimen which later turns into an unfavorable response is often misdiagnosed by well intentioned health care practitioners as "food allergies" or "allergic sensitivity." These practitioners believe that repeated exposure to certain foods will sensitize your immune system to those foods and precipitate allergic reactions which may manifest themselves in overall impaired performance. While this interpretation is not totally without merit, BioBalancing argues against it in the majority of cases and argues instead for the fact that the individual who responds in different fashion at different times to the same nutritional regimen likely possesses a cyclic acid/alkaline biochemical profile.

The biochemical mechanism underlying true allergic reactions such as those you might experience for example as a result of exposure to ragweed, pollen, molds or animal dander is generally not the same as the acid/alkaline mechanism which results in substantial impairment of physical and psychological performance. Individuals suffering from a cyclic change in acid/alkaline biochemical imbalance require not one but two or more nutritional regimens depending upon the phase of their biochemical cycle. The case history which follows will illustrate this point.

A CASE OF PREMENSTRUAL SYNDROME (PMS)

Grace was 31 years old and had been suffering from PMS for more than 17 years. Her symptoms had become progressively worse year after year since she had started having them at the age of 13. At first, as an adolescent she had complained of cramps and abdominal bloating. Medications did little to relieve her pain. Over the past few years her symptoms had become much worse and had taken a "psychological" twist. She had begun experiencing depression during the premenstrual phase of her cycle starting at the time of ovulation and deepening into "black despair" the closer she got to menstruation. With the initiation of her period she felt "drained but relieved." Upon termination of her period she felt "like a human being, but kind of scared of what's going to happen to me the next time around." Grace was told by her physician that every woman has some discomfort and that her depression was likely the result of the fact that she was perhaps a bit too "body-aware." Her physician (a woman) then proceeded to recommend a *sensitive* and nationally respected psychiatrist specializing in women's problems who would help Grace strengthen her "coping mechanisms." Astonishingly, Grace's psychiatrist (also a woman), told Grace that PMS was a "bunch of hooey" and that her depression could only be dealt with by having Grace "take a good look at (herself)" and "get in touch with (herself)." Grace went through 4 years of psychotherapy on a weekly basis. She sought out BioBalancing as a last resort.

Initially, with a venous plasma pH of 7.46 averaged over the first 14 days of her menstrual cycle, Grace proved to be a mixed metabolizer during both the menstrual phase (days 1 through 4) and the preovulatory phase (days 5 through 14). With an average pH of 7.50 during the second 14 days of her cycle, Grace proved to be quite alkaline during the premenstrual phase. The acid/alkaline evidence was clear beyond the shadow of a doubt. Grace had a very convincing case of PMS. Her PMS was decidedly not, "a bunch of hooey," as her psychiatrist had believed.

The following example describes how Grace ate on a typical day prior to initiating her program of BioBalance Therapy.

Breakfast: 1 egg, oatmeal with 2% milk, decaffeinated coffee.

Lunch: Cup of pea soup, tunafish sandwich on diet rye, tea with lemon.

Dinner: Chopped sirloin (diet lean), salad, baked potato, mixed vegetables, herbal tea.

Grace also supplemented this regimen with a full spectrum multi vitamin/mineral supplement.

If you look at the Appendix, you will see that this type of regimen is appropriate for individuals tending to metabolize in mixed fashion as Grace did from day 1 through 14 of her cycle. This regimen is however completely inappropriate for neutralization of alkaline imbalances similar to the alkaline imbalance Grace suffered from during the premenstrual phase of her cycle. In fact, because of its moderate overall alkaline inducing nature, Grace's nutritional regimen served to *accentuate* her pre-existing alkaline imbalance, thereby worsening her premenstrual symptom severity.

Accordingly, Grace was instructed to continue eating in her usual fashion from day 1 through 14. She was instructed however to eat in a fashion appropriate for alkaline types during her premenstrual phase (from day 14-15 through 28), as listed in the Appendix. An example of how she was instructed to eat during the premenstrual phase of her cycle is listed below:

Breakfast: Fresh squeezed grapefruit juice, melon, regular coffee (not decaffeinated).

Lunch: Low fat yogurt (1% or skim) with fresh fruit, regular tea with lemon.

Dinner: Chicken breast, zucchini, brown rice, herbal tea with lemon.

The supplements Grace was to take during her premenstrual phase and only during that phase are listed in the Appendix in the section dealing with alkaline types. During her premenstrual phase, Grace was also instructed to avoid some of the supplements she had been taking prior to initiating BioBalance Therapy.

Grace responded extremely well. She had the good fortune of starting the program on the 15th day of her cycle and her regimen kicked in within 24 hours. For the first time in 21 years she went through her premenstrual phase completely symptom free! Her average premenstrual pH dropped from an average alkaline high of 7.50 and stabilized in the immediate neighborhood of 7.47. To Grace's delight she also found that her premenstrual breast tenderness and bloating resulting from water retention were not part and parcel of "being a woman" as she had been told so often by well intentioned physicians and by her psychiatrist.

Grace's recovery was however not without incident. When her period began, Grace's symptoms (which usually vanished at that time) *now reemerged with a vengeance* and persisted until day 15 when her premenstrual phase reinitiated. For some reason Grace had misunderstood her instructions and mistakenly thought that the nutritional regimen appropriate for her only during the premenstrual phase of her cycle was to be adhered to throughout her entire cycle!

Consider for a moment what Grace had inadvertently done by making this error. Remember, by raising your venous plasma pH you become increasingly alkaline, whereas by reducing your venous plasma pH you become increasingly acidic. Stated in slightly different terms, you *reduce* your alkalinity by making yourself *more* acidic. If you are already acidic or relatively normal to start with, then an increase in acidity is the last thing you would want. In making her error, Grace effectively lowered her average pH during the "normal" (non premenstrual) portion of her cycle from 7.46 to 7.41. The former value is characteristic of her peak biochemical performance while the latter value is characteristic of an excessively acidic state and severely impaired performance. Grace's regimen as outlined in BioBalance Therapy as appropriate only during her premenstrual phase served to accentuate her acidity during that phase thereby reducing her pre-existing alkalinity and thus normalized her. While acidic accentuation was precisely what Grace wanted during her premenstrual phase, it was the last thing in the world she wanted during the remainder of her cycle. By mistakenly adhering to an acid-inducing regimen throughout her entire cycle, Grace neutralized her pre-existing premenstrual alkalinity *but* transformed her pre-existing mixed state which she experienced from day 1 through 15 into a severe acidic state. Consequently, she now *self-induced* a case of severe *menstrual/postmenstrual syndrome*! Fortunately, this condition was immediately corrected after Grace revised her nutritional guidelines to conform with those originally outlined in BioBalance Therapy.

Her psychiatrist who was not aware of the fact that Grace was undergoing BioBalance Therapy concluded that Grace's newly evolved symptomatology was the result of "regression" and the fact that Grace had "subconsciously" stumbled upon the "root" of her problems. Her psychiatrist believed that this so-called "root" was simply too threatening for Grace to come to grips with on her own. Given your knowledge of BioBalancing you can see that this fanciful interpretation of Grace's situation has limited merit. As it turned out, Grace simply readjusted her regimen, aborted her symptoms and terminated psychotherapy.

Grace's BioProfile before BioBalance Therapy has already been listed above. After making her error, Grace's BioProfile looked like this:

Premenstrual (day 15 through 28) pH = 7.46

Menstrual (day 1 through 4) pH = 7.41

Preovulatory (day 5 through 14) pH = 7.41

Through her error, Grace self induced menstrual and post menstrual (or preovulatory) syndrome. After correcting her error and achieving BioBalance, Grace's pH throughout her entire cycle was approximately equal to 7.47.

A final note regarding this case is appropriate at this point. It would be an error to think of the BioProfiles discussed here as being somehow representative of premenstrual syndrome *for all women* and menstrual/postmenstrual syndrome *for all women*. These BioProfiles apply only to Grace's case. Remember, as I've already stated, *individuals possess BioProfiles, diseases and impaired performance do not.*

If you're wondering whether cyclic acid/alkaline imbalances are peculiar to women, they are not. The case of Adam presented in Chapter 4 (The Feingold Diet) illustrates the fact that males can cycle as well.

VI

The Crisis in Psychotherapy

Attacking psychotherapy is a thankless task. People who have gone through psychotherapy do not want to be told that they have wasted their time and money on something which may have done little if anything to improve their condition. People who know nothing about psychotherapy generally cannot understand why anyone would want to attack a profession consisting of individuals who ostensibly want to help those who are emotionally troubled or diseased.

The psychotherapists I have met both in academia and professionally are generally well versed at verbal smoke screening and do an excellent job of deflecting attacks upon their lucrative profession. Psychotherapy, regardless of any of its so-called schools of thought is predicated upon a romantic and antiquated notion of human behavior which has historically been reinforced by popular literature and art. I hope to show you why this notion has very little to do with reality.

Before I go any further let me state emphatically that I am *not* opposed to psychology in general. There are disciplines within psychology such as theories of education and child development (among others) which deserve attention and respect. However, I draw the line at psychotherapy, that area of psychology which attempts to account for emotional disease *purely* on the basis of social and verbal interaction and without factoring human metabolism into its analyses. Trying to develop any meaningful theory or working model of psychological disease or psychopathology with disregard for BioBalancing is tantamount to trying to understand planetary motion with complete disregard for gravity!

Let me tell you a story that should put the value of psychotherapy in clearer perspective.

When I was a graduate student of psychochemistry I became suspicious of psychotherapy's attempt to relieve disease through the so-called "talking cure" or by having the patient "talk things over." I suspected that behavioral and emotional disease was in fact the result of subtle yet significant biochemical imbalances. Everytime I would question the fundamental effectiveness of psychotherapy, my colleagues and professors would engage in what I call an intellectual shell game. For those of you unfamiliar with it, the shell game played at carnivals is a slight of hand trick where a carnival performer places a pea under one of three shells or small cups, then rapidly shuffles the shells around and asks you to guess the shell under which the pea is located. If the performer is skillful, you can be fooled almost every time. In the intellectual shell game played by most psychotherapists, each so-called school of thought competing for recognition in psychotherapy becomes a shell and psychotherapy's effectiveness is the elusive pea. Let me give you only a few of the many actual examples I have run across. If you are not familiar with all the terms I'm using in these actual examples, don't worry, I'm sure you'll get the point soon enough. As a rule of thumb you may want to make note of the fact that the fancier the buzz words, the greater the psychotherapist's snow job.

If you come on strong attacking Freudian psychoanalysis as being too sexually oriented and without scientific foundation, you will be told that Sigmund Freud's views are outdated and that newer perspectives have replaced his.

If you keep hammering away and attack Rogerian therapy as being too passive, you might be told that it is incorrect to believe that Carl Rogers' views are both necessary and sufficient but that they should be supplemented with other therapeutic modalities in a more "eclectic" fashion.

If you attack cognitive theory and attribution theory as being too mentalistic, you might be told that in theory psychotherapy certainly does not rule out biological causes for emotional disease.

If you question the effectiveness of psychotherapy regardless of the school of thought being invoked and you do so by employing psychometric tests you might be told that psychometric tests are too ethnocentric or contrived and that they don't really measure what you think they might be measuring, and that only a qualified professional who is keenly atuned to his or her patient's needs, truly understands how distressed the patient really is. Psychometric tests incidentally are quantitative tests *devised by psychologists or psychiatrists* to determine the extent of emotional disease.

These evasive tactics among countless others can be summed up by a joke I once heard. The patient spills her emotions out to her psychotherapist. The therapist says the patient is distressed because she hates her mother. The patient counters by stating that she really loves her mother. The therapist tells the patient that she is wrong, and that she in fact hates her mother so intensely that she cannot face up to her intense hatred and only believes that she loves her mother. The therapist goes on to tell the patient that this type of "repression" of true emotions will require far more therapy than the therapist had originally estimated!

Sigmund Freud was quite adept at this type of snow job. Colleagues who disagreed with his psychosexual theory of behavior were told that they suffered from especially severe forms of the disorders that Freud was describing. Accordingly, Freud believed that these dissidents found his theories far too threatening and therefore they were in exceptional need of psychoanalysis! Dictatorial political regimes play a more brutal form of this game by institutionalizing political dissidents. Dictators reason that if you don't share their political ideology then you must be crazy and should be placed in a mental institution. Some physicians also play this game in that once a physician has you pegged as a "neurotic" with a "stress related" disorder then you'll never redeem yourself and get that physician to take you seriously. Some readers may have had first hand experience with this type of physician.

The type of point-counterpoint I have listed here can go on forever. You see, psychotherapists can be pretty slippery. They have become adept at snowing the opposition and smoke screening virtually any attack on any form of psychotherapy by hiding the terminally ill condition of psychotherapy under one or another so-called school of thought, thus the analogy to the shell game.

Here's how the pea beneath the psychotherapeutic shell was exposed.

A group of individuals was selected by certified psychotherapeutic experts as making good candidates for short term psychotherapy. This group was split into two subgroups. One subgroup underwent psychotherapy under the guidance of qualified psychotherapeutic experts. The other subgroup unknowingly received psychotherapy under the guidance of impostors who knew nothing at all about psychotherapy. Each of these impostors was briefly trained in the art of masquerading as a qualified psychotherapeutic expert. The dialogue below is taken verbatim from a session. I won't tell you if the exchange is between a patient and a "qualified expert" or between a patient and an imposter. I'll let you decide.

Therapist (T): "Hi, Mr. Faversham, I'm Dr. Engels. Won't you be seated please. So, what's on your mind?"

Patient (P): "Hi, I'm a little nervous, I've never been in therapy before."

T: "No sweat, just take it easy. I'm here to help. Can I get you a glass of water? If you'd like you can stretch out on the couch and relax."

P: "No thanks, I'll be all right."

T: "So what seems to be troubling you?"

P: "I don't know where to start. I guess life in general. I'm feeling tired lately, I mean really tired. Sometimes it's so bad I can hardly get out of bed and face the day. My doc says I'm ok, he says I'm stressed out and that I should get some professional advice, not that I'm crazy or anything."

T: "I'm sure you're not... crazy that is. I know what you mean about being tired, I've had days like that. Does it happen often?"

P: "Yeah, it's getting worse lately. My wife's been getting on my back about it. She calls me lazy and says I should get some help. I swear, sometimes that woman drives me nuts."

T: "Really... women, can't live with them, can't live without them." (mutual laughter).

P: "No kidding, she's on me all the time. I just feel drained."

T: "Speaking of women, talk to me about your mother."

P: "Now there's a nut case if ever I saw one. Man, that old lady really drove me nuts. 'Do this, don't do that, why can't you just finish your work and not leave everything half done. Look at your brother, he does everything on time.' Jesus, I'll bet my blood pressure goes up fifty points every time I think of her."

T: "Stress can do a nasty number on you. Sounds like your physician knows what he's talking about. Also sounds like you're having the same problems with your wife."

P: "Yeah. I mean they're cut from the same cloth... that's pretty good, I never really thought of that."

T: "That's what I'm here for, to help you sort things out."

P: "Yeah, o.k. Man, sometimes I'd like to do my wife in, I get so ticked with her. I won't or anything, but she really pushes me to the limit."

T: "Have you ever discussed your feelings with your wife?"

P: "Nah, you can't talk to her, she never listens. I'm just tired of it all. . . and listen to this . . ."

T: (interrupts) "Hold it. What's happening right now?"

P: "Whadya mean?"

T: "What did you just tell me?"

P: "I just said I'm fed up with it."

T: "What were your exact words just then?"

P: "Uh, let's see I was talking about my wife and I think I said I'm pretty tired of it, so?"

T: "Say it again."

P: "I'm pretty tired..."

T: (interrupts) "Hold it right there, what did you tell me when you first came in?"

P: "I said I'm pretty tired most of the time... you mean maybe my marriage's got something to do with this?"

T: "Look I'm not here to pass judgment on your marriage. I'm here to act as a guide and help you get in touch with your feelings. All I'm saying is that we may have hit upon something there if you feel it's important. How *you* feel is at issue here."

P: "Wow, that's kind of interesting, I've never thought of that before."

T: "Let's get back to your mom."

P: "Yeah, wow she really worked me over and my old man too. All she did was clean the house and bitch at us until the day she died. She even bitched on her death bed... (pause, starts crying). Listen I'm really sorry, I didn't mean to fall apart like that, she just died last month."

T: "Hey, no need to apologize. You obviously have some pretty strong feelings about her."

P: "I know it. The whole thing is just tough to deal with, know what I mean?"

T: "I sure do. As I said, women... can't live with them... you know the rest. Keep talking, you're doing fine. Feel any better now?"

P: "Yeah, I do. Thanks. I think I will have that glass of water."

Approximately 40 minutes later.

T: "Ok Barry, I see our time for this session has just about run out. I don't want to interrupt but I'd like to summarize what I think happened today and give you some food for thought for our next session. It's pretty clear that you've got some unresolved feelings about your mother. Obviously you care a great deal for her but there are things that went unsaid between the two of you before she died. Somehow you're repeating this pattern with your wife. I see a lot of anger that's being held back and a lot of love too. I think if we can let that pent up anger out constructively, we might get you back on track and get the depression under control. Why don't you give some thought to what happened here and schedule another session with my secretary. By the way, if you're interested, there are a some good books and articles I can suggest that deal with your problem. If you have the time, you may want to look them over. They might give you some insights into your problems and if you want, we can discuss them in the course of our discussions. Any questions?"

P: "No. I think maybe I'd like to read those books. Listen, thanks for your time. I really feel like we're onto something. How long do you think this will take, I mean before I get in touch with this thing so I won't be so tired anymore?"

T: "That's hard to say. Everybody's different. Keep that in mind. We'll have to take it a step at a time."

P: "Sounds good. Thanks. So long."

T: "See you next week."

To make a long story short, individuals in each subgroup were asked to evaluate both their therapists and their progress at the end of a three month period. Here are the results.

1. The individuals receiving treatment from the impostors reported feeling somewhat *better* than the individuals receiving treatment from the certified experts.

2. After three months of "intensive" therapy, no one in either of the two subgroups reported that his or her distress was adequately resolved.

3. Perhaps of greater significance is the fact that the impostors were ranked higher than the experts in such categories as apparent intelligence, insight, ability to sympathize and empathize.

This experiment is suggestive of the fact that the benefits an individual will derive from psychotherapy as conducted by a "certified expert" are no greater than the benefits derived from a discussion with a confidant.

You can see then why I cringed when an acquaintance recently stated that she wanted to try BioBalance Therapy, fearing that if she went to a qualified psychotherapist and that if the therapist erred in the course of treatment, she might suffer irreparable damage to her psyche. Don't laugh, this statement was made by an extremely bright young woman suffering severe depression. Her depression incidentally was relieved within one week after she initiated a program of BioBalancing. Her statement reflects the remarkable stranglehold the psychotherapeutic community has upon how most of us think and view ourselves. Needless to say, many so-called experts have hotly contested the significance of this study. Here are some of their reactions:

"Of course the patients being treated by the impostors felt better, the impostors were inept and could not get the patient to focus on the root of the problem which if exposed would have proven very threatening to the patient." I think the experts are saying *you've got to feel worse before you feel better* (sound familiar?).

"Of course the patients liked the impostors more than the qualified professionals. The professionals made their patients work hard to get to the root of their problems. It's not easy to like a person who makes you dig up unpleasant experiences. The impostors just told their patients anything they wanted to hear." I think the experts are saying *if you want to feel better, go to an imposter but if you want to feel worse then go see an expert.*

"Three months worth of therapy may not be conclusive, sometimes therapy takes a lifetime." I think the experts are saying *they haven't the foggiest clue as to how therapy will evolve and that it could be open ended.*

"It's important for the patient to *believe* that the person administering the therapy is 'in the know' otherwise the therapy will not be taken seriously." I think the experts are saying that *fraudulent practice is absolutely critical to psychotherapy's success and that if psychotherapy is exposed for what it is, it won't work* (assuming of course that it works in the first place).

In light of what I've said thus far, my next statement may really shock you.

As far as I'm concerned the problem with psychotherapy is that there is not enough of it!

I say this because I feel that no matter how well BioBalanced people may be, it would be criminal to stop them from seeking others to talk with albeit for a fee in times of distress. Hence, I would propose that our society *deregulate* psychotherapy and allow anyone who wishes to promote himself or herself as a professional talker/listener to hang a shingle up and go into business!

Is there any precedent for the type of *deregulation* which I propose? It turns out that in ancient Greece, individuals would hire the services of professional mourners at wakes and funerals. Professional mourners would cry and carry on during funerals to elicit and draw out grief from friends and relatives of the deceased. The process of letting go of your feelings in this fashion is known as *catharsis*. Friends and relatives of the deceased *knew* that the mourners were acting out, yet they also felt that the mourners were performing an important service. Analogously, our society should allow the operation of professional talkers/listeners with minimal if any government regulation.

If the entire business of "talking things over" were deregulated, the cost of psychotherapy would likely drop precipitously. Assume for a moment that you suddenly felt the compelling need to "talk things over." Assume you had a choice of spending $20 per hour talking to someone who came highly recommended by friends as empathetic, compassionate, witty, articulate, intelligent, and possessing great insight or $125 per hour talking to a "certified expert." How would you choose?

Incidentally, Barry Faversham was later brought into BioBalance. As you may have guessed, neither his mother nor his wife made any appreciable contribution to his depression and exhaustion. Mr. Faversham was excessively acidic. His fruit and low fat yogurt breakfasts were sapping him of his strength. It took him approximately three weeks to regain his energy and vitality.

Let me recast the confrontation between BioBalance Therapy and psychotherapy as follows. We humans consist of a "word processing" component and a "food processing" component. Psychotherapy would like for you to believe that emotional disease is the result of a malfunction of your word/symbol/cognition processor. BioBalance Therapy recognizes that social/verbal/linguistic events as mediated by your "word processor" may have a profound impact upon short term emotional well being. BioBalance Therapy however views most emotional disease as the manifestation of a malfunction of your "food processor" regardless of whether the initial cause was social or nutritional. Furthermore, BioBalance Therapy realizes that in cases of substantial biochemical malfunction, all of the talking to all of the world's most qualified experts may not do much good.

People having the most difficult time understanding this are individuals who suffer from "situation specific" disorders such as phobias. When I talk about this, someone will say, "But I don't understand how BioBalancing applies to me. After all, while I can't say that I feel all that well most of the time, I don't have a panic episode unless I am in an elevator, or driving a car across a bridge, or driving a car on a limited access highway, or if I'm in a small confined space, or if I feel trapped in one way or another." I'll discuss a specific case regarding the impact of BioBalancing upon phobic response later.

Some psychotherapists may diagnose panic disorders among others as "stress related." However, once again it must be emphasized that your ability to withstand stress or *your threshold of tolerance to stress is tied to how well BioBalanced you are*. Individuals who are not BioBalanced will typically shatter on contact whereas individuals who are BioBalanced will demonstrate resiliency and will flexibly bend under pressure. It's quite common for individuals to state that they can handle far more stress after being BioBalanced than before. Let me give you a specific example.

Ellen, a stock broker suffering from "nerves and anxiety" recently underwent BioBalance Therapy. Ellen used to suffer from insomnia and spend nights pacing the floor worrying about the stock market. Seven years of psychotherapy did nothing for her. After being BioBalanced, Ellen not only felt well, but continued feeling well even after the October '87 stock market crash where some of her clients reported record financial losses. She reported that she didn't lose her mind over the crisis but simply did "what had to be done." This is what I would call the mark of a "psychologically" strong person. Interestingly enough, after completing her program of BioBalancing Ellen's psychotherapist (unaware that her client had engaged in BioBalance Therapy) told Ellen that she seemed "so well-centered" and that she seemed better able to "cope." Well, she was! However, her "coping mechanisms" were fortified as the result of a change in her eating patterns as determined by her program of BioBalancing and not as the result of "talking things over" with her psychotherapist for seven years. Anecdotally, Ellen made an interesting observation. "I'm convinced that America and the rest of the world is facing a severe economic downturn. What will the American public, now spending almost *half a trillion dollars* per year on medical care do when unemployment hits all time highs? Why doesn't somebody make BioBalance available to the public *now* as a low cost effective alternative? I really fear that we're headed for some very hard times if this alternative to conventional medical care isn't instituted quickly." Irrespective of whether financial collapse is imminent, I'm forced to agree with Ellen's conclusions regarding the runaway cost of health care and its impact upon both our health and the economic health of America and the world.

I've already given you an example of how "food processing" can influence "word processing." In the case of Adam, the hyperkinetic child, Adam's school work improved significantly after he achieved BioBalance. He did so without the benefit of coaching or environmental "enrichment." His mother, a developmental psychologist, was at first understandably mystified.

Let me say one other thing about stress before I continue and that is that while stress may very well contribute to panic or to emotional disease in general, diagnoses involving stress are rapidly being grossly abused by the medical establishment. BioBalancing recognizes that *life is stress*. BioBalance Therapy cannot cure anyone of life. No doubt, stress probably contributes to all types of disorders. Conversely undergoing "stress management therapy" via one or another form of the so-called "talking cure" or "relaxation therapy" may well contribute to emotional restabilization. Yet the intelligent person must ask, "how much does stress contribute to my condition and conversely, to what extent will stress management help?." The contribution made to emotional restabilization by therapies involving "stress management" and "relaxation" pales to insignificance compared to the contribution made by BioBalance Therapy. Focusing much of your attention upon "stress management" and "relaxation" and expecting these forms of therapy to appreciably contribute to your long term recovery is equivalent to believing that rearranging the deck chairs on the Titanic would have delayed its sinking.

The entire issue of stress has been carried to ridiculous lengths by both the medical/psychotherapeutic community and by a gullible public. Recently an acquaintance of mine was diagnosed as having a "stress related disorder" by her physician and she was advised to seek out assistance from any one of a number of *qualified* mental health practitioners who specialized in stress management. It turned out that the patient's condition was soon correctly diagnosed by another physician as terminal cancer. The first physician would still not back off from her diagnosis and went on to state that stress undoubtedly contributed to the cancerous growth. What amazed me was the fact that the patient's family believed her! The patient's family consisted of bright, well-educated individuals who never bothered to ask the physician how she knew that stress had anything at all to do with cancer. This story is doubly tragic in that it demonstrates the stranglehold the medical and psychotherapeutic profession have on how the public views itself and disease.

If by now you're thinking that perhaps the impact of BioBalancing goes far beyond psychotherapy and overlaps medicine in general, you're absolutely right. A successful physician recently underwent BioBalance Therapy for suicidal depression. He had of course tried all types of nutritional and behavioral therapies to no avail. He had also spent many years and a small fortune on various methods of psychotherapy. He achieved BioBalance within a period of two weeks, felt exuberant and made a rather insightful statement.

His observation, *"BIOBALANCING IS SO EFFECTIVE THAT ANY MEDICAL DIAGNOSIS OR PROCEDURE CONDUCTED WITH DISREGARD FOR THE PATIENT'S ACID/ALKALINE BIOCHEMISTRY IS OF NECESSITY INCOMPLETE AND IS PROBABLY VERY FAR FROM COMPLETE."*

This physician is in essence telling you that unless you are also being BioBalanced, you are NEVER going to get your money's worth from your physician. Think about it.

Let me summarize the problem with psychotherapy and the medical profession's view of psychology and the human condition. When my daughter Jenni was four years old she was doing some card tricks. Prior to the completion of each trick she would say some magic words such as "abracadabra." I asked her if she believed that the words made the magic. She paused pensively and blurted out laughing, "Daddy, that's silly. The magic's in the cards, not in the words!" I never ceased to be amazed that the psychotherapeutic and medical establishment cannot understand something that was obvious to my (then) four year old daughter.

Unfortunately, psychotherapy has shaped the way most people think and sadly it has done a great deal to confuse and mislead the public and camouflage the underlying causes of disease. To make matters even worse, many social circles consider it chic and a sign of superior intellect to spice up conversation with psychotherapeutic jargon. Over the years I have seen how many individuals view themselves psychologically. Let me give you some examples.

The Cave Man School of Psychonutrition

(Many men I know subscribe to this way of thinking) "Food has nothing to do with it. It's all will power and in the mind. BioBalance is for women, fat people and crazy people. We real men know who we are and no hot dog or granola bar is going to mess us up!"

The Naughty and Nice School of Psychonutrition

(Virtually every dietician I know subscribes to this way of thinking). "Spare ribs are a naughty naughty. Coffee's a naughty naughty. Sugar's a naught naughty. Low fat yogurt's nice. Whole grains are nice. Pasta salad's nice. Vitamins and minerals are nice provided that we take them SENSIBLY. When WHOLESOME, SENSIBLE and WELL BALANCED nutrition fails then... psychotherapy's nice provided of course that it's conducted by a 'certified' expert."

Almost There

"I'm sure that BioBalancing works for most people but it will never work for me. I'm just too complex to be helped by something as simple as food. My problems can only be solved by a 'certified' psychotherapist."

Being There

"While BioBalancing is not everything, it is a substantial part of the food-mood-health puzzle. Psychotherapy is no better and no worse than talking to a confidant. Any sensitive, intelligent and caring person is qualified to be a psychotherapist."

I repeat: *"ANY MEDICAL DIAGNOSIS OR PROCEDURE CON-DUCTED WITH DISREGARD FOR YOUR ACID/ALKALINE BIOCHEM-ISTRY IS OF NECESSITY INCOMPLETE AND WILL TYPICALLY BE VERY FAR FROM COMPLETE. IN FACT ANY MEDICAL PROCEDURE OR DIAGNOSIS CONDUCTED WITH DISREGARD TO YOUR ACID/ ALKALINE BIOCHEMISTRY CAN BE AS DANGEROUS AS RECEIVING A TRANSFUSION WITH DISREGARD TO YOUR BLOOD TYPE."*

"IF YOU ARE NOT BIOBALANCED, YOUR PHYSICAL AND PSYCHOLOGICAL WELL-BEING WILL LIKELY BE SUBSTANTIALLY IMPAIRED."

These last two statements are quite provocative. Many individuals report that after being BioBalanced and viewing medicine and psychotherapy in this fashion, nothing is really quite the same again. They say that while the concept underlying BioBalancing is quite simple they nonetheless get quite frustrated in their attempts to communicate that concept. Most of the people these individuals talk to think that BioBalancing has little to do with getting well and that recovery from so-called psychiatric disorders results from "power of suggestion" or that it's all "in the mind" (sound familiar?). Other people don't understand that BioBalancing is radically different from other forms of nutrition or medicine and they will state that they too are seeing one type or another of "wonderful" physician or nutritionist. Still others become hostile when it is suggested that their problem has anything to do with faulty metabolism. At the conclusion of a seminar I recently gave, I told a persistent young woman that if she really believed that BioBalancing was not for her then she must be an extraterrestrial in that her biochemistry was not carbon based! She could not see the humor in my statement.

If you undertake a program of BioBalance Therapy you will soon discover that your new found way of thinking is not shared by most people around you. Some may even choose to believe that you are troubled. During prehistoric times, our ancestors attributed the type of disease to which I refer in this book, to the influence of the evil eye. If they became diseased they would seek out the assistance of a witch doctor. Today most people believe that if they feel psychologically "together" and "centered" it is because they have been permitted to do so as the result of psychotherapeutic assistance or because they have "well integrated" personalities and adaptive "coping mechanisms" (fancy psychotherapeutic buzz words). This rather romantic notion of psychological health is so ingrained that even some people who have successfully undergone BioBalance Therapy cannot disabuse themselves of these illusions.

Indeed, one psychotherapist who succeeded in ridding himself of panic episodes through BioBalance Therapy was unwilling to alter his practice because he felt that some disease best lent itself to the so-called talking cure administered (of course) only by a certified expert such as himself. I can only imagine the thoughts he entertained, "Heaven forbid if the public's psyche were placed into the hands of an unqualified imposter masquerading as a qualified expert!" In any case, the rationalizations this psychotherapist invoked in justifying the continuation of his practice even after he had seen the light of day would probably make your head spin.

I heard somewhere that you can go a lifetime without sex, but that you can't go more than five minutes without at least three or four really juicy rationalizations. Truer words were never spoken. Tragically, because of ignorance and apathy many people would rather curse the darkness than light a candle and undergo BioBalancing. Some of the examples and case histories which follow will give you a better idea of what I'm talking about. Let me rephrase the shortcomings of psychotherapy by reviewing what I've just said from a different perspective.

Recently I appeared as a guest speaker on a radio talk show. The show's hostess was open-minded, but sympathetic to psychotherapy. She found it difficult to believe that BioBalancing could reverse disorders that she and tens of millions of individuals believed could only be altered by long hours of "talking it through" with a certified professional. She openly admitted that she had spent a good amount of time in psychotherapy. She went right to the heart of the matter by asking me if too acid or too alkaline a biochemical condition was all there was to human nature. "Dr. Wiley," she asked, "are we just as simple as that? I mean, is being too acid or too alkaline all there is to it?" I emphatically replied that human beings are far more complex than that, but I immediately went on to state that deeper levels of complexity would not lend themselves to being unraveled in a psychotherapist's office. She was understandably puzzled and continued probing. "But after all, doesn't psychotherapy plumb the depths of the human mind?." I responded by telling her that this is precisely what the profession, along with the movie and television industry would like for you to believe. In actual fact, the most sensitive and qualified psychotherapist doesn't know any more about what makes you tick than a plumber or auto mechanic. Having studied psychochemistry, I'm not kidding when I make that statement. Not only is there no evidence that psychotherapy is effective, the evidence I've seen strongly argues that psychotherapy is worth as much as a good heart-to-heart talk with a confidant. There is also a growing literature within psychology supporting these views, especially when it comes to the accuracy of psychological diagnosis.

Needless to say, people balk when I say this. Usually (when I give a seminar) there is at least one individual in the audience who will jump up and angrily defend psychotherapy by remarking that he or she was a mess and was helped substantially after going through psychotherapy. I always counter a remark of this nature by asking what that proves. If you take the defense of psychotherapy at face value you'll see that it is meaningless. After subjecting psychotherapy to the same type of scrutiny to which I have subjected BioBalancing and other forms of nutritional therapy, I have found that the level of confidence associated with the statement, "Psychotherapy works," is almost zero. The results are appalling. The comparison becomes more extreme when we compare actual recovery rates of the two therapies. Recovery is almost always achieved *and maintained* through BioBalancing in less than four months. With psychotherapy, oftentimes *no results* materialize within time frames *exceeding* ten years of analysis.

There are however some individuals who do feel better after a course of psychotherapy. I do not believe that "it's all in their minds." They *do* feel better. However, with statistics as poor as these, any intelligent person is forced to wonder if improvement *during* psychotherapy can be attributed *to* psychotherapy or to something else. More often than not, after some probing, the individual who claims to have derived benefits from psychotherapy will (sheepishly) admit that he or she changed dietary habits to lose weight (as is usually the case) and thereby increase self-esteem. In many such cases, it turns out that the weight reduction diet was more appropriate to that person's biochemical type than previous diets, thus resulting in inadvertent psychological benefits. "Talking it over" had virtually nothing to do with full or partial recovery.

Sometimes an individual will defiantly and triumphantly tell me that no dietary modifications were engaged in, thus implying that he or she was the exception to the BioBalance rule. As I will show you later, people who have invested a good deal of time, money and emotion in psychotherapy will defend it with fanaticism. It is highly likely given the odds, that biological factors come into play when individuals get well during psychotherapy even if no dietary changes are made. Some individuals, for example, suffering transient or temporary candidiasis (systemic yeast infections) which manifest themselves as psychological disturbances will spontaneously recover regardless of how much they might "talk things over." Such cases are especially prevalent with women after childbirth, miscarriage, abortion, frequent casual sexual encounters or a protracted course of antibiotics or steroids. It is simply an illusion to believe that psychological problems are "deep-seated" requiring a good deal of "sensitive" probing by a "certified" psychotherapist.

Does all this mean that I believe that human beings need no longer engage in social interactions and merely eat appropriately in order to achieve and maintain a state of BioBalance? Not at all. I do not doubt for one moment that "talking things over" does indeed help... for a while. Compassion and concern are very important, if not critical, to individuals and to the future of humankind. Sadly, the world is woefully lacking in compassion.

Unlike science which has one primary school of thought, psychotherapy probably has more schools of thought than there are psychotherapists. Our judicial system is becoming painfully aware of this fact. That's why "expert" psychiatric testimony is becoming less and less valued in courts of law. You might wonder what all of these schools of thought have in common. After all, they all seem so different. The common thread connecting these various schools of thought consists of the assumption that psychological disease is somehow *learned*. I am sure that there will be many psychotherapists who will ardently disagree with this statement. But don't be fooled by the language they may use in trying to overturn it. They may tell you that psychological problems are part of a "process of complex socialization" or that they result from "poor ego defenses" or "poorly integrated coping mechanisms" or "dislocated family dynamics" or "psychosocial trauma" or "excessive stress"...and the list goes on and on. All of these fancy academic phrases really boil down to one key word and that word is *learning*. Somehow, somewhere along the line psychotherapists will argue that you have *learned* to experience the world around you in diseased fashion because you have been consciously or subconsciously *taught* to do so by parents, peers, friends, family, associates, social stimuli, political events, etc.

As you are about to find out, this last statement, while not completely untrue, must be qualified to the point where it is virtually meaningless. I say this because even in cases where a singular and clearly-defined traumatic event precipitates or causes acute psychological distress or disease, it is possible to reverse that distress by readjusting or literally realigning an individual's biochemical structure through BioBalancing. What I'm saying may sound pretty fantastic and counterintuitive at first. I'm actually telling you two key facts: (1) Social interaction or social conditioning does not primarily contribute to psychological disease. A combination of genetically-inherited faulty metabolism/biochemistry and inappropriate nutrition (as defined within the context of BioBalancing) contribute primarily to psychological disease. Psychological disease is not *learned* in the overwhelming majority of cases. (2) Verbal interchange has little long term value in the wake or aftermath of social stress. In such cases where psychological disease has in fact been learned or caused by traumatic social events, it is not necessary to "talk things over" for prolonged periods of time (in some cases perhaps a lifetime) in order to *unlearn* that disease. As astounding and counterintuitive as it may seem, one can literally eat one's way out of psychological disease *regardless of the nature of its cause!*

Most people don't find the first statement too difficult to accept. Many people however, find the second statement very difficult to accept.

It's pretty much like telling people in the middle ages that the earth revolves around the sun. Surely, you would have been thought insane to believe that. Just go outside and see for yourself. Can't you see the sun *rise* in the east and *set* in the west? You must be crazy not to be able to see the sun move, how could you possibly believe that the sun is stationary and the earth moves?

Similarly, isn't it obvious that if psychological disease is brought about by verbal or social cues (i.e., it is *learned*) then you should be able to be talked out of it?

Let me be more specific in making my point. Let's say you're generally feeling O.K. You board a plane and in flight it undergoes total engine failure at 35,000 feet and begins an uncontrolled descent. You're gripped with fear. At 10,000 feet the engines resume functioning and the plane makes an emergency landing. You get off, shaken, and find it impossible to board another plane again. In fact, you probably start having nightmares and you become anxiety prone throughout the day. Things may get so bad that friends tell you that you probably need psychotherapy. How, you may ask, could food possibly have anything to do with this? Clearly a problem such as this must have been learned. After all, you were doing reasonably well before your flight and you developed problems as a result of a scrape with what appeared to be imminent death. "Come on," you're thinking, "I can't believe that eating peas and carrots and not eating tuna fish is going to change anything here!"

Let me ask you this. If I forced you to get on a plane what would happen? You'd probably panic. Let's say I sedated you or had you drink liquor prior to your boarding a plane. What do you suppose would happen? People who have gone through precisely this type of trauma and later resorted to drugs or alcohol on a subsequent flight reported feeling spaced out, giddy, drunk, and had almost complete disregard for whether the plane crashed or not. Amazing... how could a pill and/or liquor or more generally a chemical, change your feelings about an event that *you learned to fear*? They can. Your biochemistry has been altered to the point where the negative associations coupled with the plane (fear of flying) have to some extent been defused and have lost their impact.

I've often seen psychotherapists rationalize the use of medications by telling a patient that the medication will enable that patient to better come to grips with a hidden or repressed fear which will in the long run be unearthed by "talking things over." It should become increasingly apparent to you by now that this rationalization is complete and utter nonsense. No doubt if you are afraid of flying and if I medicate you heavily or give you several stiff drinks you may lose that fear but not without experiencing a number of undesirable side effects. Let's carry this example a bit further. Is it possible to create a medication which will restructure your biochemistry so that you can feel good about resuming air travel *without* any side effects? Does that really sound so incredibly farfetched? Having come this far with my book you've no doubt already realized that the "medication" I'm talking about is food, as *defined within the context of BioBalancing*.

I don't for a minute doubt that getting used to air travel through a gradual programmatic reintroduction to flying will help to a limited extent. *Relearning* not to fear air travel (in this case) forms part of a type of psychotherapy which is (understandably) called *Behavior Modification Therapy* and which has its academic roots in a school of psychological thought known as *learning theory*. Relaxation therapy is incidentally another form of behavior modification therapy. I must however hasten to add that the efficacy of any such program is largely determined by whether an individual is achieving BioBalance. In summary, the probability of your deriving any significant benefits from a program of behavior modification depends substantially upon how close you are to being in BioBalance prior to the time you start the program. Indeed, in many cases, achieving BioBalance is *sufficient* to resolve the problem without the use of any type of program involving behavior modification therapy. Conversely, in many cases, programs of behavior modification without BioBalancing fall short of the mark and provide little if any relief.

Think of your biochemistry or metabolism as a spooled watch spring. This analogy is not really different than the analogy of the "floaters," "sinkers" and "gliders" I gave earlier in this book. Every individual has a certain setpoint or point of equilibrium and because of genetic factors, the stiffness of your biochemical spring will determine how that spring will oscillate back and forth about the center of equilibrium. When your spring is in equilibrium you are feeling pretty well. The further from equilibrium your spring is stretched, the greater the extent of your psychological distress, disease or disorder. What causes your spring to oscillate? Primarily genetic make-up and nutrition where the latter is defined within the context of BioBalancing. I would be lying if I told you that social events did not affect your biochemical balance. Yet, it is critical to keep things in perspective. If you go into a socially stressful situation in a state of relative biochemical imbalance, then you will likely emerge in a state of severe imbalance. If your metabolic or biochemical spring is mildly distorted and you board the plane, that spring will become severely distorted. To make matters worse, if the foods you eat are not completely appropriate for your metabolic or biochemical type, regardless of how "wonderful" and "wholesome" they may be, that disequilibration caused by the near crash will *not be corrected in any reasonably brief time frame by talking things over*. You can talk and talk and talk and talk until you turn blue in the face and your biochemical spring will simply remain unbalanced, as long as your diet remains inappropriate.

Did you ever wonder why in a crisis situation such as the one which I cited in the example I just gave, some individuals will emerge as emotional wrecks over long periods of time, some will be emotionally impaired over shorter time frames, others will be emotionally bruised, while others still will emerge relatively unscathed. Psychotherapy attempts to explain this variation in terms of "coping mechanisms" which are formed during childhood and are shaped by various social interactions. While this attempted explanation sounds reasonable at first glance, it doesn't hold water because there is little correlation between your social background and how you will respond to stress *if you don't factor BioBalancing into the equation*. Let's say for example that you emerged emotionally crippled from the near crash I have used in the example and that you went to see a psychotherapist. The issues your psychotherapist may find significant might relate to your being an only child or the middle child, or a male among males, or a female among females, or the first-born, or the last-born, or an ethnic minority, or your having had an overbearing mother, or your having had an overprotective mother, or your having had a submissive father, or your having had a domineering father, or... you can fill in the rest. If you want a "social hypothesis" to explain away psychological disease and you have the money and the time I'm sure that you'll be able to find a *certified* psychotherapist who will make the events fit the hypothesis.

A friend of mine who owns a clothing store used to tell the following joke in showing how good a salesman he was. One day he had only white suits in stock. A customer walked in, tried one on and liked the fit, but stated that he wanted a blue suit. My friend yelled to his associate in the back room, "Turn on the blue lights, the man wants a blue suit!" The same story holds for psychotherapy. Sooner or later somebody will confabulate enough of a story to make it look like it's the right fit... but don't be fooled, it's just the blue light! In fact, as soon as you leave the psychotherapist's office, chances are that you are going to relapse again and again. Even Sigmund Freud knew about this type of relapse and called this phenomenon *the slow return of the repressed*. In the light of day, its still a white suit!

There are so many theories of psychological disease that it would be impossible and pointless to discuss them all. One however merits further discussion only because it is in vogue today. It is called attribution theory. Fully 75% of the individuals who undergo BioBalancing have undergone psychotherapy. They reveal that their psychotherapists are practicing some form of attribution theory although they don't call it by this name.

Attribution theory postulates that you feel the way you do because of how you *interpret* your bodily sensations. Specifically attribution theory claims that you *attribute* your emotions to your bodily sensations. Attribution theory has as its roots the old chicken and egg argument that psychiatrists and psychologists have been playing with for centuries, namely does the mind cause body or does the body cause mind? Let me give you an example. A female client with premenstrual syndrome seeking assistance through BioBalancing reported feeling borderline psychotic symptoms prior to her period. She also reported feeling bloated, having breast tenderness and experiencing vague muscular pains. The attribution theorist/psychotherapist that she had gone to see prior to seeking assistance through BioBalancing told her, "It's O.K. to have those feelings before your period, most women have them, you're just a little too *body aware*. You're paying a little too much attention to your body." What the psychotherapist doesn't realize is that it isn't the woman's awareness that's *causing* her to experience the disabling psychological symptoms, it's her biochemical imbalance which is being manifested *simultaneously* as a psychological problem and as a somatic or bodily problem as well. The "body awareness" ploy is very popular and is used frequently by physicians and psychotherapists in attempting to talk individuals out of a disorder, usually women with a disorder called mitral valve prolapse. You may remember I have mentioned mitral valve prolapse in dealing with case histories earlier in this book. Incidentally, some physicians love to play at being psychotherapists since between 75% and 90% of the complaints they hear daily have no basis in anything they learned in medical school. Don't be surprised. Physicians receive nominal training in nutrition and zero training in BioBalancing. A patient, usually female, with a prolapsed mitral valve will state that her heart is skipping beats and sometimes will race for no apparent reason. She will likely be told, "You're just a little too *cardiac-aware*. Why don't you forget it, go out and live your life." This is not an easy task if your heart is galloping away at 220 beats per minute and skipping beats continuously. The psychotherapist or physician is trying to talk the patient into the following fantasy: if she gets her "mind" off her body, then she'll be O.K. It would be laughable if so many people were not suffering from this guilt-inducing bogus approach to problems the medical and psychotherapeutic establishment cannot deal with successfully.

Attribution theorists jokingly like to summarize attribution theory by telling the public the following story. The dog wakes up and wonders how he feels. He looks over his back and sees his tail wagging, so he concludes that he must be happy. I like to describe attribution theory a bit differently.

When I was a child in the 1950s, the comedian Sid Caesar had a weekly variety show on television. One of my favorite characters that Sid would portray was the absent-minded German professor, complete with strange accent, floppy top hat, disheveled tie and cutaway coat. One night the professor was being interviewed regarding his theory of pain:

Interviewer (I): "Professor, tell us about your theory of pain."

Professor(P): "Vell, you zee, it's dis vay. Ven zeh brhain zees zeh painvul act it rhegisters pain, und you veel it, yah?! Vat, zeh brhain can't zee you don't veel."

I: "So Professor, according to your theory, if I take this sledgehammer and smack your thumb while your mind is on something else, then there will be no pain."

P: Zats right! Zo, now vee trhy it, yah?" The Professor places his hand on a block, turns to the audience and starts whistling. The interviewer proceeds to smack the professor's thumb with the hammer. The Professor stops whistling immediately and stares out into space but doesn't acknowledge the pain actively.

I: "Well, Professor, how do you feel?"

P: (Obviously straining to his limits). "Vondervull! Und now I vill inshpect zeh thumb."

The Professor lifts his hand which has been outfitted with a fake plastic oversized black thumb.

P: "Zeh brhain vill now look dirhectly at zeh thumb."

The Professor looks and begins screaming.

P: "Yah, zeh pain, I can veel it… yaow, does zat hoit!"

Just think of it, millions of people lining up to be told that they're O.K. They're only a little too aware of their bodies and that's why they're diseased. The old absent-minded professor would be proud. What started out as a joke has ended up as mainstream psychotherapeutic dogma.

Some of BioBalancing's clients openly admit that they were raised in the real world equivalent of Mr. Rogers' Neighborhood and they are still emotional wrecks. Of course, their psychotherapists tell them that their idyllic childhood ill prepared them for life. More "blue light" therapy!

By now if you've been closely following what I've been saying, you might wonder whether it's possible to reverse BioBalancing and actually induce severe disease in individuals who are otherwise feeling well. *The answer is yes.* In fact, I've already given you a few examples. I'll give you another more dramatic example shortly.

Fifty years ago schizophrenia, manic depression, conversion hysteria, and many other disorders were all considered "mental"/"social" disorders. Today they are more commonly acknowledged as being bio-chemical in nature. Why stop there? Why not draw the line to include mild depression and mild fatigue? Why not draw the line to include a "mild case of nerves?" Why not draw the line to include "coffee nerves?" Why not draw the line to include *feeling well*? Why not draw the line to include feeling fantastic or possibly even beyond?

In summary, while you can learn about morals and ethics, while you can learn about the theory of relativity, while you can learn about BioBalancing, while you can learn to play a musical instrument, while you can learn to tap dance, etc., you just can't learn to be chronically depressed and fatigued, you can't learn to be schizophrenic, you can't learn to be chronically anxious, you can't learn to have panic attacks, you can't learn to have premenstrual syndrome, you can't learn to have "undiagnosable" bodily pains and discomfort. However, BioBalancing and learning are interrelated as I have already shown you with Adam's case history (Chapter 4) in that cognitive and intellectual performance will in many cases improve when an individual achieves BioBalance.

VII

The Refugees of Psychotherapy

In Chapter 4, I listed a number of different nutritional therapies currently being promoted in the popular marketplace and I gave you examples of how each therapy failed. As I've already mentioned, there are many schools of psychotherapy. Consequently, it would be futile for me to recount to you a case history for each psychotherapeutic school of thought. Instead, I'll present some case histories where it might otherwise have been concluded that the patient's problems would not have been influenced by BioBalancing.

YOU TAKE CARE OF MY BODY, I'LL TAKE CARE OF MY MIND

Joanna was 29 years old and 20 pounds overweight. She had suffered severe depression in her late teens and had attempted suicide. Since that time she had been in psychotherapy on a weekly basis.

"Actually I'm not here for my depression" she said, "I'm here to lose weight. My friend went through with BioBalancing and lost more than 90 pounds painlessly. I'm involved in a fast-track administrative job and I've just got to look my best. I'm also working out at the local Nautilus so I might as well get my body together with the best nutrition around."

Joanna was asked why she felt BioBalance Therapy could come up with a diet that could differentiate her psychological problems from her physiological problems and work only on the latter. What she said was interesting but not novel.

"You know, I'm tough. I've been to hell and back. I've had some pretty hairy things happen to me in my life and I've had to work through a lot of these experiences and it's made me all the tougher. I got suicidally

97

depressed about ten years ago and I almost killed myself. But I found a really great psychotherapist and I'm working it out. I'll never, and I mean never, get back to that state of depression again. So that's why I'm here, to get my body together and not my head. I might also build up a little more self esteem if I slim down, but my self esteem is already pretty good. I've got a really good handle on who I am, O.K?… so let's get started."

Joanna's train of logic is pretty standard for most individuals who think that somehow they can hold on to who they are or fix onto their identity regardless of the type of biochemical changes they may undergo. Most people like Joanna think that their sense of identity is somehow tied to realizations they have made of themselves in the past in counseling or psychotherapy. This view surprises me to some extent, especially in light of well publicized results of experiments conducted by the government regarding the effects of hallucinogenic drugs like LSD on personnel. These studies suggest that even small quantities of hallucinogens can precipitate radical personality changes within minutes. Some changes were so severe that unwitting subjects committed suicide, subjects who were judged as possessing remarkable psychological strength and who might have been regarded as model citizens. It's no mystery that a cardinal rule of military intelligence is, 'don't ever let them capture you alive'… regardless of how strong you may believe your convictions and will power to be. Given the degree to which you can be overwhelmed by psychochemical interrogation, it's only a matter of time before you'll tell the enemy everything. While the impact of acid/alkaline nutrition is not as pronounced as that of the major hallucinogens, it can nonetheless be rather dramatic. It all makes you wonder. At any rate, I'll demonstrate my point to you insofar as Joanna was concerned.

Joanna got off to a good start. She proved to be modestly acidic. It turns out that she did in fact change her eating habits to lose weight two years after initiating psychotherapy. The eating habits she adopted were more appropriate for her biochemical type. At that time low carbohydrate diets for weight loss were in vogue. It was clear that this dietary change and not psychotherapy was responsible for her "getting a handle on herself" as she put it. Her response to BioBalancing was predictable. She began to lose weight but not for long. She kept straying from her diet. She became a bit upset with the program.

"My psychotherapist says that I'm self-destructive and that's why I keep cheating on my diet. She says more psychotherapy should help me work things out. I suppose she's right." Joanna was then asked if she wanted to be cured of her so-called self-destructive impulses.

"Sure." she responded with a laugh. "What is this some kind of quack hypnotherapy or something?"

She was told that BioBalance Therapy was neither quackery or hypnotherapy, but she was also told the real probable cause of her suicidal depression ten years ago was her diet. She was told that it was a change in her diet and not psychotherapy that caused her to get a handle on herself. She was very skeptical. It was explained, though certainly not recommended, that if she were to completely reverse the dietary guidelines given to her as part of her program of BioBalance Therapy, she would see the profound influence of food on her life. Cheating a little on her BioBalance regimen as she had was child's play. A complete reversal and she would find herself feeling as severely depressed as she was 10 years ago. Joanna felt she had been challenged. It didn't take long before disaster struck. She showed up at her next consultation seven days later looking very disheveled.

"I'm really hanging on. I'm really hanging on." She pursed her lips and began crying. She recovered her composure. "I keep telling myself it's only the food. But, and this is so scary, I'm not sure I believe that anymore. Like, I know it's not true but yesterday I thought maybe, just maybe... I said I'd never do that again, but the thoughts are coming back. I've spent ten years getting a handle on this, I can't believe I could lose it all in one week. How can it be food? Maybe it's just me."

It was clear that emergency measures were in order. Joanna was put on a regimen designed to rapidly enable her to achieve BioBalance. One week later Joanna was her new found self again.

"That was really frightening! What the hell is going on here? I spend ten years getting my head together and a change in my diet blows it away in one week. I met with my psychotherapist last week when I was really screwed up. She and I talked things over. She said I was regressing. I told her it was my diet and she suggested I be committed for inpatient treatment at the psychiatric center. I said it really was the food and she thought I was paranoid. This is kind of scary. But it's all so strange. It's like the past ten years of psychotherapy were wasted. Man does that ever blow me away."

FEAR OF FLYING AND OTHER PHOBIAS

Muriel was 50 years old, fat and phobic. Her views regarding phobias and psychological disorders were not unlike the views held by most people who've had no exposure to BioBalancing. Muriel's life prior to the onset of her phobias was relatively free of chronic problems that would be classified as psychological. At the age of 25 Muriel's life took a turn for the worse when she was almost killed in a plane crash. The incident (which I used as an example earlier in this book) involved her being aboard a passenger plane which had engine failure in mid-flight and almost crashed. The plane's engines reignited at low altitude and the plane underwent an emergency landing. Several people aboard were seriously injured. Muriel escaped with no physical injuries. Consequently, Muriel became phobic of air travel and avoided it for the next 25 years.

She also began having nightmares and would oftentimes begin to feel "strange" (as she put it). Curiously, the mild premenstrual syndrome which she experienced prior to her near crash also began to intensify and began expanding to other phases of her menstrual cycle. She began skipping periods in her late 20s with some periods as many as 60 days apart. Her gynecologist (a man) had suggested that she undergo a hysterectomy at the age of 30. He told Muriel that her symptoms were probably caused by hormonal problems and that a hysterectomy would likely bring relief. As Muriel stated it, "The real nightmare began after the hysterectomy because my symptoms didn't go away and I gained 80 pounds in no time flat. My gynecologist said that it was impossible for me to still feel phobic since the hysterectomy he performed had done away with the hormonal problem causing the phobias. He said I was becoming a fat hypochondriac and that my postoperative phobias were now all in my mind. He said that if I let things get out of hand he would have to suggest that my husband Roger have me institutionalized. I was devastated because I wanted so badly to get well and I had also always wanted to have a child. I realized then that I could do neither. That's when I started seeing a psychotherapist. I figured that my problem was not hormonal since the hysterectomy didn't help so I probably needed a psychotherapist for a deep-rooted mental problem. Not that I'm crazy or anything. (Sound familiar?). Anyway, my phobias began to generalize. That's the word my psychotherapist uses. She's such a wonderful person, I've been seeing her for about eight years. You see, I'm developing new phobias." Muriel had lots of them. "I can't drive across a bridge. I can't ride in an elevator. If I can't get my jewelry off easily I get panicky. If the zipper of my blouse or dress or skirt gets stuck I get panicky. I'm even getting panicky if I can't take my nail polish or wedding ring off. My psychotherapist says that my marriage is the cause of all this. She says I'm feeling trapped and that's why I'm getting panicky. She says when I started therapy that this will need a great deal of talking through to achieve resolution, yes I think that's how she put it."

The correlation between Muriel's PMS prior to her hysterectomy and her phobias was pointed out to Muriel during her initial consultation through the use of the "spring" analogy I've already used. Muriel looked puzzled and could not see the connection between her near plane crash, her expanding and worsening premenstrual syndrome, her phobias, her hysterectomy and her weight management problem. In fact, after she recovered from her crying bout while talking about her inability to have a biological child, she grew a bit indignant.

"Well… now… I for one don't see what all this has to do with my being here. I'm a realist and I know that nutrition can't undo my fear of flying or my other phobias. I'm working on that with my psychotherapist. I'm here because a friend of mine said BioBalancing might be able to help me with my weight problem. I for one am a firm believer in good, wholesome nutrition. So that's why I'm here."

If you recall what I said earlier in this chapter, you'll understand the illogic of Muriel's assumptions and conclusions. Some people who go through BioBalancing want to understand the ramifications of BioBalancing. Muriel was clearly not one of them. She had compartmentalized the universe into neat little categories. Some problems she believed required sensitive probing by a certified expert while others required wholesome and wonderful nutrition. Muriel's beliefs went unchallenged.

It turned out that Muriel was significantly alkaline and possessed a systemic yeast infection as well. Her recent dietary changes towards a diet richer in protein because as Muriel stated, "Everybody knows that protein is good for you", accentuated her alkaline imbalance and likely caused her phobia of flying to generalize. It was also reasonable to conclude that prior to her hysterectomy she was slightly alkaline during the menstrual and preovulatory phases of her cycle (days 1-14) and very alkaline during the premenstrual phase. This oscillation in acid/ alkaline imbalance was probably accentuated by the psychological shock she experienced as a result of her near crash while flying. As you will now understand, Muriel's hysterectomy and psychotherapy did her about as much good as having her palm read.

Approximately eight months after initiation of her program of BioBalancing and for the first time in her adult life, Muriel achieved her ideal weight. Muriel had painlessly lost 50 pounds. Her recovery from her generalized phobias was also rapid, far more rapid than expected given the amount of time she had spent in psychological distress. It turns out there is no correlation between rate and extent of recovery on the one hand and symptom severity or duration on the other. I'm not certain yet why this is so. In any event, Muriel still did not see any connection between her generalized phobias and her weight problem. What really surprised Muriel, however, was something which happened three months after being brought into BioBalance. For the first time in 25 years she boarded a plane. She flew from New York City to Florida and back without tranquilizers or alcohol. She was amazed.

"I told a professor of psychology at the local stress center about BioBalancing and he said that it was quackery... all quackery. He said the only reason my phobias got better was because of power of suggestion. He said that my weight loss was probably also power of suggestion too. He said people like me get phobic because we get too aware of our bodies (sound familiar?) and we associate muscle tension and increased heartbeat with anxiety and fear and that's when we panic. He said I had to learn how to manage my stress. Now I for one must admit that he's got a point... even though, I must admit that I do feel wonderful!" Muriel was hopeless. "I just can't believe this! I just feel wonderful! But how on earth could BioBalancing cure my fear of flying? I mean, I didn't imagine that near crash I had 25 years ago. I suppose finally my psychotherapy must have kicked in. Well, I'm sure both my psychotherapy and those wonderfully BioBalanced foods helped."

Muriel wasn't disabused of her fantasy. Then Muriel said something that was surprising because people like Muriel generally don't see the connection between their disease and anyone else's problems. They generally believe that while they had a problem which was resolved through the use of BioBalancing, the next person with a similar problem probably needs a psychotherapist! "Now I think I'll suggest that my husband Roger come along and try the BioBalance diet too. He's been so tired and cranky lately. Can he be helped? Is there a diet to help people who are cranky and tired?"

Muriel was told that there was no such thing as the anti-cranky diet. She was told that if her husband's problems were due to a biochemical imbalance as they likely were, then he too should try BioBalance Therapy.

Muriel understated Roger's condition when she called him cranky. Roger's conversation on the phone redefined the word hostility. Roger kicked off his monologue on the telephone with some rather descriptive verbal abuse. "QUACK! If I had only known that BioBalancing wasn't administered by *real* doctors I would never have *allowed* my wife to go through with it! QUACK! It's all quackery! Do you know that my insurance company won't reimburse me one penny! Not one penny! QUACK!... QUACK!"

People never cease to amaze me. Muriel had by her admission spent more than $30,000 for medical care. Recall, she underwent a hysterectomy at the age of 30 which prevented her from having children. Robert S. Mendelsohn, M.D. in his book *Confessions of a Medical Heretic* calls such elective surgical procedures "ritual mutilations" at the hands (no doubt) of a *qualified* gynecologist. Roger thought of all the money he had gotten back from insurance, probably 80% of the money that he had paid for Muriel's medical care. Still his 20% and yearly deductibles added up to a handsome amount. I can't tell you the number of times people have refused to undergo BioBalancing because of the fear of not being reimbursed by insurance but continued to be operated upon and talked to by *certified, sensitive experts.*

Roger and people like him remind me of another joke told by my friend, I mentioned earlier, who owned a clothing store and joked about the white suit. A store owner sometimes slashed prices on really awful looking and poorly made clothes. When a customer would try a suit on and remark at how awful it looked the salesman would respond, "For a price like this, who cares about the fit!" Then he'd ring up another sale. I guess some people like Roger just can't resist a bargain!

The Hunt for Red October

In his best selling novel *The Hunt for Red October*, Tom Clancy graphically describes life aboard a nuclear powered attack submarine against a backdrop of geopolitical tension and international intrigue. In reading this book it is clear that the world's navies, especially submarine fleets rely primarily upon the ears of their sonar crews. In an underwater world where visibility is typically nonexistent, rapid and precise recognition of underwater sound patterns by highly skilled sonar operators aboard a submarine can mean the difference between life and death.

Doug served as a sonar operator on board a nuclear powered ballistic missile submarine, known in the jargon as a 'Boomer.' He took a great deal of pride in his work until he snapped. "I used to be gung ho. My work was always a challenge and I enjoyed it. I know there's a morbid side to it if you think about the destructive capability of our boat, but I was brought up believing that we had to defend ourselves and that the other side was up to no good. Man, it got so I was so well tuned to sounds that I could tell what crews were on board enemy boats. Ever read 'Red October'? Let me tell you, the sonar dude Jonesy in that book had nothing on me. But that was then and now is now. I don't know what happened, I just fell apart one day. We were under the polar ice cap just listening. I'd done it before but this time something was different. I was really keyed up trying to get a fix on some noise off in the stern sector when it suddenly dawned on me that the noise was a group of incoming torpedoes. Somehow I knew they weren't torpedoes but I just freaked. I sat there knowing we were deep underwater and under ice, and my head just kept telling me that the noise I picked up was inbound and that we weren't gonna live a hell of a lot longer. Man, I started sweating bullets. All I could think of were the torpedoes punching holes in our hull and the boat just imploding under all that pressure. And then, and I'm not sure I can describe this, everything around me in the boat looked like it was part of a fast forward video even though I knew that everyone was relaxed and I was the only one who was about to flip out. I just couldn't keep my cool. I wanted to scream "Incoming!", but I just froze. The funny thing is that a part of me knew there was no threat, but I just kept freaking. Finally the boat's doc gave me some tranks (tranquilizers) and suggested that I be given some R & R (rest and recreation), but I knew that my number was up. Funny thing about it was that I knew from that moment on that I'd never be the same. I just had to get off the boat or I'd go nuts."

"That's when I started seeing shrinks. I spent two years talking about everything. And I mean everything. My sex life, my mom and dad, my feelings about war, about life and death, my being adopted and not knowing who my biological folks were, about my being a dove in hawk's clothing, I mean it just kept going and going (sound familiar?). You know, I kept telling these guys that I thought maybe there was something wrong with my body, but they just kept coming back at me and kept telling me that all the test results were normal and that I kept insisting that there was something wrong with my body because I wanted something to be wrong with my body and because I couldn't face up to the fact that *I* was the problem (sound familiar?). Listen, I'm no dummy, I got a Bachelor's in engineering and I took some psych courses in college. I took enough psych to wonder where these shrinks get their ideas. But man, I was hurting so bad and I was on so many drugs to keep me from freaking out that I was ready to believe anything. I got electric shock therapy too. Blew half my damn memory away for a while. You know, that's not fair man, that's sort of like brain washing. It's sort of like interrogation. They want you to see it their way because if you don't, they tell you that you're crazier than they first thought. Sounds like the movie *One Flew Over the Cuckoo's Nest*, you know that nurse Wretched, she wasn't playing with a full deck and neither are these shrinks. I thought only the Gestapo or the KGB put people in the nut house when they vote the wrong way, but man our shrinks are doin' the same thing! Anyway, I just know that this thing is some kind of biochemical problem and I know there's gotta be a better way to pull out of this."

Doug was right. Here's a description of how Doug ate on the submarine.

"O.K. I was really into a body building trip. Lifting weights. So I thought I'd build myself up with lots of protein. That's the neat thing about serving on a boomer, the food perks are out of sight. Ham and eggs, steaks, the works. I just couldn't get enough, and it showed, man I was in real fighting form."

It showed all right, but in more ways than one. Doug was still working out and sticking to his "cave man" diet of red meat and reduced carbohydrate intake. His muscles were clearly pumped up... and so was his venous plasma pH, peaking out at 7.51, a substantial alkaline high. Doug may have been a submariner but his metabolism was in orbit. It was little wonder that Doug could barely keep it together. Under similar metabolic circumstances it's my guess that Admiral Rickover, father of the U.S. nuclear navy, would have felt exactly as Doug did. Doug was somewhat amused by the dietary recommendations he was told to abide by to achieve BioBalance. "Wow, vegetarianism. Low fat yogurt and sprouts. Wimp food. Sounds interesting. Just grains, fruits and veggies for a month and then a little low fat dairy. Hey, I mean sure, I'll try anything if it works."

Within six weeks Doug found that he could substantially reduce his medication. By the end of a three month period, Doug had stopped taking all of his medication and reported that he was symptom free for the first time in more than three years.

"Listen, this stuff is great. No more shrinks. I feel like I'm back in the world of the living. Man was that ever weird. I didn't even tell my shrink what was going on. I just dropped out. Those guys'll never understand anything. Hey! Let me lay this one on ya. I won this greyhound dog in a poker game, she's great, I called her Boomer, can you dig that? Her old show name used to be Zero because she couldn't run to save her life. So just for kicks I put her on my diet. Man, that baby just took off like a bat out of hell. Her skin cleared up too. She used to have these awful pimples and acne on her chin. A dog with acne, can you believe that! Listen I'd bet there's big bucks in this with race horses and dogs, man you could make a killing!"

Perhaps Doug had a point. At any rate, it was good to see that he was finally out of the "depths" metabolically and back on terra firma.

VIII

Questions Most Frequently
Asked About BioBalance Therapy

Question(Q): *I've read lots of books on health and sometimes I see my problems as part of a case history. I didn't recognize my symptoms in any of the case histories here. How do I know that BioBalancing will help me?*

Answer(A): If you're asking this question you've missed the whole point of this book. Simply try it. BioBalancing's not just for people whose symptoms resemble the case histories in this book. BioBalancing is for everyone!

Q: *How can I determine my acid/alkaline biochemical profile and how do I go about correcting any imbalances?*

A: Read the next chapter.

Q: *Should I attempt to eliminate my acid/alkaline imbalance under the supervision of a physician?*

A: In their book, *Psychodietetics*, Drs. Ringsdorf and Cheraskin (both M.D.s) state that even well trained mainstream physicians only know a little more about nutrition than their receptionists.

Typically physicians practicing within the mainstream will make one of the three following comments regarding BioBalancing:

1. Venous plasma pH never changes. Anyone who tells you that diet can change venous plasma pH is a quack.

2. Venous plasma pH is always changing. Anyone who tells you that he or she can determine the impact of diet upon that change is a quack.

3. Diet doesn't affect much of anything except for your weight. Anyone who tells you that your diet has a significant impact on mental health is a quack.

There are some enlightened physicians who would take issue with these statements based upon their personal clinical experience. These physicians may be able to assist you.

In order to obtain a list of physicians who may be receptive to BioBalance Therapy, contact:

> The American Holistic Medical Association
> 41011 Lake Boon Trail Suite 3201
> Raleigh, NC 27607
> (919) 787-0116

For a fee the American Holistic Medical Association (AHMA) will provide you with a booklet listing the names, addresses and telephone numbers of health care professional nationwide and internationally who bias their practices in favor of a holistic approach to medicine. *Incidentally, I am not implying that the AHMA endorses BioBalancing Therapy.* I am speculating that on average, member health care professionals of the AHMA may be more willing to assist you than more orthodox allopathic physicians.

Q: *If I'm on medication for a psychiatric or physical disorder how do I get off that medication?*

A: You need not discontinue medication to engage in BioBalance Therapy. After achieving BioBalance it is likely you will start feeling better. You may choose to tell your physician that you are feeling better and that you would like to work with him or her and phase out or reduce your dosage of medication.

Q: *What effects do medications have upon acid/alkaline biochemistry?*

A: It's been my observation that many medications, especially psycho-pharmacological agents affect the central nervous system and do not substantially alter acid/alkaline biochemistry. In essence, many psycho-pharmacological medications blind your central nervous system to any acid/alkaline storms that might otherwise be raging.

Q: *What effects do viral or bacterial infections that result in common types of disease such as colds or flues have on acid/alkaline biochemistry?*

A: Relatively common opportunistic diseases generally accentuate an underlying acid/alkaline imbalance.

Q: *In your article published by the International Journal of Biosocial Research (see references) you talk about the possible impact of BioBalance Therapy upon disorders other than those that are commonly diagnosed as psychogenic. Some of these disorders are commonly referred to as "dread" diseases such as cancer. Have you had any experience in dealing with AIDS? Would you speculate about the impact of BioBalance upon AIDS?*

A: In answer to the first question, no. I have had no experience in assisting individuals with AIDS. In answer to the second question, if I had AIDS I'd certainly try BioBalancing. I would speculate that BioBalancing would not interfere with any other type of medication or therapeutic modality.

Q: *Why should physicians, or for that matter, why should anyone believe you as opposed to anyone else?*

A: I would suggest that you carefully read Chapter 10 and my article as published by the *International Journal of Biosocial Research.*

Q: *Why venous blood? Why not saliva pH or the pH of any other bodily secretion?*

A: Let me again answer this very important question. Only venous blood returns from sites of cellular activity. The relative acid/alkaline imbalance of venous blood (its pH) is therefore an excellent indicator of the efficiency of molecular/ion transfer and exchange which occurs at the cellular level.

Venous plasma pH is regulated in part by the coenzyme matrix that drives both the Embden-Meyerhoff and Kreb's metabolic cycles. The overall efficiency of these cycles can be determined mathematically through the use of reaction diffusion rate kinetics which also describe the evolution of chemorhythmic cycles, cycles which have recently become the focus of great deal of attention in the field of psychochemistry. The formalism I briefly mention here is mathematically complex and a more detailed explanation would far exceed the scope of this book. Saliva, urine, feces, arterial blood, lymph, tear or lachrymal secretion, skin, nails, hair and other secretions provide no such measure. These bodily secretions periodically fall into and out of vogue with various factions of the alternative health care community and the lay public. Currently, it would appear that saliva is being "rediscovered." All I can say is that after 20 years of careful observation and research, it is clear that only venous blood provides a reliable indication of the molecular transfer taking place at the cellular level. All other indicators may be deceptive and unreliable.

Q: *How frequently must venous plasma pH be measured? Does a measurement schedule appropriate for men differ for women?*

A: The schedules for both men and women are given in detail in the next chapter.

Q: *Have the nutritional regimens outlined herein been computer analyzed for nutritional adequacy? Doesn't BioBalance Therapy focus only on venous plasma pH to the exclusion of everything else and therefore aren't individuals who undergo BioBalance Therapy at risk for severe malnutrition of one kind or another?*

A: Let me answer this question with another question. Whom do you propose should computer analyze BioBalancing? The phrase "computer analysis" conjures up high tech images. Let me remind you of the "GIGO" rule of computer programming, namely that Garbage Input yields Garbage Output. If the computer algorithm uses "the four basic food groups philosophy" as the basic constraint... then BioBalancing will fail the test (surely this does not surprise you). If the computer algorithm uses a high carbohydrate, low fat constraint... then BioBalancing will fail that test too (surely this does not surprise you either). What test could you use then? If you look at my observations as published by the *International Journal of Biosocial Research* (see references) you'll see that BioBalance Therapy is successful in assisting approximately 90% of a given population... a population that was independently analyzed as being psychologically and physically distressed.

You might feel that the one year observation period I used is too short. In that regard you may be correct, however I should hasten to point out that twenty year follow-ups with various metabolic types indicate that recovery can be sustained without any deleterious side effects. This point is worth emphasizing insofar as acidic types are concerned since acidic types must eat high protein, low carbohydrate regimens indefinitely. These regimens have recently fallen into disfavor with physicians, dieticians and nutritionists. I've repeatedly stated that BioBalancing is not an "either/or" form of therapy. Now you might feel that twenty years is not a sufficient time period to justify your attempting BioBalancing. If this is your objection, then I'd have to ask you what your alternatives are? You could muddle along waiting for the certified experts to give their benediction to BioBalancing. If you're waiting for that kind of recognition you may well wind up waiting a long time.

Q: *I see in the Appendix that iron is contraindicated for certain metabolic types, namely acidics. Isn't iron deprivation dangerous? What if an acidic type suffers from iron deficiency, will that deficiency magically correct itself after that individual achieves BioBalance?*

A: Let me start by correcting you. Iron is not contraindicated for anyone. Supplemental iron taken in therapeutic doses is contraindicated for acidic types. Should a physician prescribe iron for an acidic individual if that individual is iron deficient? I've seen iron therapy administered in this fashion and the outcome has typically been unfavorable in that the patient reports feeling worse (irrespective of the type of iron being used) and despite the fact that iron count will actually increase. The nutritional regimen appropriate for acidic types is very rich in iron and consequently corrects iron deficiency if it exists and allows the patient to achieve BioBalance. Many anemic acidic types who undergo BioBalance Therapy will report feeling a decrease in symptom severity after achieving BioBalance without the aid of supplemental iron. Once again, BioBalancing is not an "either/or" situation.

A similar situation is also true regarding calcium. Alkaline types are discouraged from taking supplemental therapeutic doses of calcium. This has caused considerable consternation among women especially in light of the current "calciumosteoporosis" alarm/craze. Note I didn't say that alkaline women should eat a calcium free diet. Sunlight, vitamin D, folic acid, calcium rich foods and anaerobic exercise will do far more to reduce an alkaline woman's risk of incurring osteoporosis than will a high potency calcium supplement which will militate against her achieving BioBalance and will likely cause her to fall short of realizing her full biochemical potential.

I should also point out as I discuss in additional detail in the following chapter, that many individuals simply cannot tolerate supplements of any nature. These individuals are advised against taking supplements altogether and are directed to rely upon more stringent counter-effecting variations of their nutritional regimens to achieve and maintain BioBalance. I suspect that this intolerance results from gastrointestinal inability to absorb and assimilate supplements of any variety. Needless to say, virtually all medically-accepted gastrointestinal tests will result in a "within normal limits" verdict. Incidentally, holistic physicians believe that insufficient hydrochloric acid secretion is responsible for this intolerance. I have discovered that this is generally not true. It is my belief that the ideal way to take supplements is sublingually (under the tongue) as is currently being done with B12. Unfortunately, I have not been able to convince any supplement manufacturer to produce all supplements in this fashion. BioBalance Therapy is simply not "high volume" enough to warrant this type of manufacturing effort.

All of this incidentally should lead you to wonder about the validity of biochemical measures used by the medical profession in defining "normalcy." I've already shown you that the accepted medical measure used to define normal pH is in fact representative of a pathologically acidic state.

Q: *Who can guide me through a course of BioBalance Therapy? Will Dr. Wiley help me through his firm, BioBalance Services?*

A: I provide a list of resources in the next chapter. Regrettably, I no longer serve the public directly. My consulting firm, BioBalance Services consults only with health care professionals in the matter of data interpretation.

I no longer deal with the public for the following reasons. I spent a substantial portion of the past twenty years gathering data and assisting individuals *pro bono* as part of a long-term, self-financed research effort. Accordingly, acquiring an understanding of acid/alkaline metabolism has long been my avocation. As public recognition grew I became deluged with requests for assistance. Consequently I began charging a fee for my time. Sadly, complex legislation regarding medical malpractice and skyrocketing insurance rates, combined with some individuals' desire for both a "quick fix" and maximum insurance reimbursement created prohibitive operating costs, and endless administrative headaches.

Q: *After I get into BioBalance, will I then be able to eat like a "regular person"?*

A: That all depends upon how you define a "regular person." To be honest with you, the answer is *no* unless you were a mixed metabolic type to start with and the root of your problem was candidiasis or an inappropriate dietary regimen. Chances are that you have been genetically programmed to metabolize foods in a deviant fashion. Unlike a course of medication where you stop taking that medication after you get well, BioBalancing is for life. Remember, BioBalancing is not a cure but is instead a method of control. If you stay on the BioBalance course you will likely reap substantial benefits. If you deviate from that course you may be deleteriously impacted.

Q: *Will my acid/alkaline profile ever change?*

A: The following milestones are significant in a person's life in terms of coinciding with possible changes in acid/alkaline biochemistry.

1. The onset of puberty.
2. The cessation of substantial physical growth (18 to 22 years of age).
3. Pregnancy.
4. Abortion.
5. Childbirth. — Incidentally, acid/alkaline disturbances afflicting mothers after childbirth (and *not* psychological factors) are almost invariably the cause of postpartum psychosis.
6. Cessation of lactation.
7. Menopause.

Q: *Speaking of pregnancy, can toxemia be correlated with a specific biochemical type?*

A: I have seen toxemia corrected nutritionally. I feel it may be correlated with excessive alkalinity.

Q: *How will I know if my acid/alkaline profile has changed?*

A: If you've been on a regimen or regimens which has/have agreed with you and then you experience the reemergence of those problems which initially caused you to seek assistance. Please note that mild transient illnesses such as colds, flues, fevers, etc. do not necessarily indicate a reversal in acid/alkaline imbalance although it is noteworthy that individuals who are in acid/alkaline balance generally report becoming ill less frequently than individuals who are not.

Q: *What is the effect of drug addiction on pH? How about cocaine and alcohol?*

A: I have not had the financial resources to pursue the impact of BioBalancing on drug and alcohol addiction. However, I feel that the impact of BioBalancing on human health in general suggests that acid/alkaline imbalances contribute substantially to drug and alcohol addictions. Additional research is warranted.

Q: *What's the impact of the different amino acids and fatty acids upon venous plasma pH?*

A: I haven't had time to fully research this. As I've said, all the research I've done thus far has has been conducted without any outside funding. Accordingly, amino and fatty acid research has had to take a back seat to other research. You should treat any and all claims regarding the impact of amino and fatty acids upon health in the same fashion that you should now be treating claims regarding the impact of foods and supplements upon health. For example, claims that certain amino and fatty acids are energy boosters, or good for women with PMS, effective in treating sleep disorders, or appropriate for championship athletes should be regarded with suspicion and as potentially bogus. The key question is, "How does a particular amino acid impact venous plasma pH?"

Q: *You spend a lot of time discussing the impact of BioBalancing upon the so-called psychiatric disorders. Why does this book's title imply that BioBalancing has an effect upon the food-mood-health puzzle?*

A: If you read my article published in the *International Journal of Biosocial Research* you'll see why.

Q: *How do I find out if I have candida?*

A: Obtain a blood analysis for the presence of candida antibodies. (NOTE: I do not subscribe to the notion that candida resides in the blood. However, a high level of antibodies indicates a response to a systemic yeast infection.) Your physician may not subscribe to this theory and therefore may not cooperate. Physicians who generally go by the title of holistic physicians may. I've already shown you how to contact these physicians.

Q: *How do I treat candidiasis?*

A: Read the next chapter in this book.

Q: *If I've got a history of feeling poorly and my spouse does too, is it a foregone conclusion that my children will share our problems?*

A: Yes, it is likely that your children will inherit some degree of bio-chemical imbalance. However, your biology will not commit you to a life sentence of feeling poorly if you take countermeasures to neutralize your biochemical imbalances through BioBalancing and do the same for your children.

Q: *Is the method of treating children the same as that for treating adults?*

A: Yes, but don't force children into radically changing their dietary habits quickly. Common sense should dictate that they will likely become rebellious. Try to ease them into the regimen(s) appropriate for them. You don't need a psychotherapist to figure out how to do this, just use common sense.

Q: *If I'm acidic won't the high fat and high cholesterol diet appropriate for me increase the probability of my getting colon cancer or cardiovascular disease even though I may feel well in the process?*

A: BioBalancing is not an "either/or" situation where you're trading off physiological well-being for psychological well-being or vice versa. You are burning off blood sugar and dietary fat at a very rapid rate if you are acidic, and subsequently you will need that type of diet to buffer you biochemically.

Q: *Is there a correlation between symptoms and various biochemical profiles?*

A: Very few such generalizations can be made. Most diabetics are very alkaline. As I've already stated, toxemia during pregnancy is indicative of alkalosis. Most individuals with elevated cholesterol, triglycerides and low density lipids are usually alkaline although a few are mixed. Most individuals with gout are alkaline, although a few are mixed. All individuals who are hypoglycemic are acidic by definition. I must reemphasize that if you have been told that you suffer the so-called *classic* hypoglycemic symptoms then there is no conclusion you can draw regarding your BioProfile. People who exhibit these so-called *classic* hypoglycemic symptoms may possess *any* BioProfile for the reasons I've discussed repeatedly in this book. Adhering to a diet appropriate for acidics because a well intentioned physician may have told you that you are hypoglycemic, could result in disaster if your symptoms are caused by a severe alkaline imbalance. Many people who believe they are hypoglycemic are not, irrespective of what they have been told by well intentioned health care practitioners.

You may find the following true story sadly amusing as I did. The president of a local chapter of the Hypoglycemia Foundation initiated a program of BioBalance Therapy. It was discovered that she was extremely alkaline and therefore not hypoglycemic. She insisted that she had to be hypoglycemic because she had the so-called *classic symptoms* and because she was an expert on hypoglycemia and had counseled people on the illness for more than 30 years. To make a long story short, she terminated her program despite the fact that she was making a rapid recovery because she was positive that her BioProfile was incorrect!

Q: *If I am hypoglycemic and therefore a true acidic type do I have to eat six or seven meals per day?*

A: No. The reason physicians recommend that hypoglycemics eat frequently is that these physicians have not devised a diet suitable for buffering the hypoglycemic's tendency to drift toward the acid end of the acid/alkaline scale. The diet appropriate for acidic types should be adequate so that three meals per day should suffice. One or two small snacks may be eaten if you feel a need for them.

Q: *What about food allergies?*

A: Most people who are BioBalanced do not have food allergies. If you are in BioBalance then I would suspect that the probability of your suffering from food allergies is low. Conversely, if you're not in BioBalance that probability is higher.

Q: *Is it possible that my acid/alkaline biochemical profile will change radically in random fashion?*

A: Excellent question. No, it is highly unlikely. If it does, you are in serious trouble and it will be difficult to neutralize these changes as they arise. The fact that you may suffer "unpredictable mood swings" in all likelihood does *not* mean you are shifting metabolic gears randomly.

Q: *How will I know if my acid/alkaline biochemistry changes during various parts of my menstrual cycle?*

A: If you're not relying on actual biochemical assays then only trial and error will allow you to make this determination. Typically you will feel well on one regimen during one phase of your cycle and you will suddenly feel poorly on that same regimen during another phase of your cycle. Should this occur, immediately switch to the mirror-image regimen (see the Appendix). Should you quickly recover and then feel poorly during that same phase from this nutritional change, then mix or blend the two dietary regimens as suggested in the next chapter. Some sample "food-mood" diaries which I have included in this book in the following chapter should give you an idea of what I'm talking about.

Q: *If I am always in BioBalance, will that guarantee that I will feel great all the time?*

A: No. Candida may disrupt your well-being if you're not careful. Other health problems may also. I will discuss more about candida control in the next chapter. Candida overgrowth is exacerbated through improper nutrition or the use of antibiotics or steroids. Social stress may also cause you to react adversely. BioBalancing will not make you "monoemotional." You will experience a broad range of emotions depending upon the social circumstance. It is unlikely that you will experience psychological disease for no apparent external cause or reason. Clearly if a terrorist puts a gun to your head and tells you that you are being held captive, no amount of BioBalancing will cause you to feel well. However the manner in which you react to your life experiences will, to a significant extent, be determined by your pre-existing biochemical stability.

Q: *What do I do if BioBalancing doesn't work for me?*

A: There is approximately a 55% probability that you will experience full recovery. There is approximately a 35% probability that you will experience a significant if not substantial reduction of symptom severity. There is approximately a 10% probability that nothing will happen. In the last case try to find a physician who will prescribe medication best suited for you with as few side effects as possible. If you fall in the 10% category do not assume that your problem is of a psychological nature and that you need the services of a psychiatrist or psychotherapist.

There are still some unanswered questions regarding BioBalancing and human physiology. However, there is every reason to believe that some as yet undetected biological aberration is the culprit, *not* a deep-seated psychological trauma.

Q: *What should I do about additives and preservatives?*

A: More and more additives and preservatives are daily proven to be harmful to human health. Although they may not be the culprits Dr. Feingold would have us believe, to be on the safe side it is wise to try to avoid additives and preservatives to the best of your ability. There is one additive that I would avoid completely, and that is *monosodium glutamate* or *MSG* There are simply too many people who react adversely to this additive.

Q: *Won't simply going on a low carbohydrate diet get rid of a systemic yeast infection?*

A: Not necessarily. Furthermore, if you happen to be fundamentally alkaline, going on a low carbohydrate diet could wreak havoc on your acid/alkaline biochemistry and accentuate your biochemical dysfunction or imbalance.

Q: *What about eating at a restaurant?*

A: If you are relatively acidic, or you have a mixed metabolic profile, then eating at a restaurant should be fairly straightforward. It is relatively simple to select a meal which will conform to your optimal dietary guidelines. If you are alkaline you should be careful to avoid greasy, salty and fatty foods. Generally, lean pork or light fish is standard fare at most restaurants. If you are ordering light fish for example, you should specify that it not be laden with butter and salt as is generally the case, since you may suffer an adverse reaction if the fish is accompanied by a creamy and/or buttery sauce.

Q: *What if I just read a good health and fitness magazine, take vitamins and minerals and eat "sensibly." Won't that be O.K?*

A: Unfortunately, if you're asking a question like this then you've missed the point I've tried to make. I would suggest that you re-read this book. By now you should understand that there is no such thing as *sensible* eating for everyone, just as there is no such thing as a well-balanced vitamin/mineral supplement for everyone. There is nothing wrong with health and fitness magazines. They have done a good deal to increase public awareness. However if you try to treat your symptoms nutritionally by using conventional wisdom which is often printed in the popular press with complete disregard for your acid/alkaline biochemical type, chances are you will fall very far short of the desired mark.

Q: *Shouldn't I just listen to my body and eat what it's telling me to eat?*

A: Do so at your own risk. Most people have poor biochemical instincts.

Q: *Can't a good nutritionist tell me what to eat? Why do I need to go through all this BioBalance stuff?*

A: If you want a lecture on the four basic food groups and you want to be told that all supplemental vitamins and minerals taken in moderation are probably good for you, then go to a nutritionist. If you don't feel that your optimal well-being is worth the time and effort it takes to determine your BioProfile then you've sold yourself short.

Q: *I've noted in the Appendix that the nutritional regimens appropriate for alkaline types include coffee. Isn't coffee really a drug and therefore bad for you?*

A: Everything is a drug in that all things have specific chemical structures. Filet of sole and spinach are drugs too. BioBalancing attempts to show you how to use foods to maximize your psychological and physiological well-being. I recommend that some alkaline individuals rely upon coffee to a modest if not nominal extent and view it primarily as a medication. Diets appropriate for alkaline individuals are by no stretch of the imagination high coffee diets. If you drink a great deal of coffee, chances are it will deplete you of vital nutrients in the long term. I have never suggested that any individual, regardless of how alkaline he or she might be, partake of a high coffee diet. Generally even severely alkaline individuals will, upon recovery, find that one cup or less of regular coffee per day is enough to stimulate and normalize their metabolic profile.

Q: *Don't all women need iron and calcium?*

A: In a way I've already answered this question, but let me answer it now from a different perspective. Yes, but in different doses. Women who are alkaline need more *supplemental* iron than women who are not. Women who are acidic need more *supplemental* calcium than women who are not. Women who shunt from one end of the acid/alkaline scale to another should be pulsed with different vitamin-mineral supplements accordingly. Women who are alkaline and who are at high risk of developing osteoporosis should increase their intake of calcium-rich foods which are not contraindicated for their metabolic type. After they achieve BioBalance, it is suggested that they gradually begin introducing supplemental calcium. More often than not as I've already stated, too high a supplemental dosage of calcium will resurrect pre-existing distress for an alkaline type. "Too high" a supplemental dose may be defined as ranging from 250 mgs to 1500 mgs per day. As you will note from the Appendix, supplemental calcium is contraindicated for alkaline individuals. Women who are alkaline and who insist upon taking supplemental calcium, should gradually increase their daily supplemental calcium intake by 250 milligrams each month. Far more importantly, they should immediately stop increasing their calcium intake if they observe any adverse reactions such as reemergence of symptoms for which they originally sought assistance.

Q: *Can't I just take a pill or shot to make my biochemistry normal, why BioBalancing?*

A: To date there is no solution as simple and straightforward as that.

Q: *What if my problem is truly mental or a problem of attitude. Then isn't BioBalancing a waste of time in my case?*

A: If you're asking this question then you've missed the point of this book. I suggest that you reread it.

Q: *Why can't I just treat my symptoms by eating foods or taking vitamin and mineral supplements appropriate for those symptoms? For example, use vitamin B-6 and stop drinking coffee for PMS; take the amino acid trypto-phane for insomnia; take calcium for muscle cramps and so forth?*

A: If you are asking this question, you have missed the point that I have been trying to make. I would suggest that you reread the previous chapters in this book. Treating disorders in this fashion as generally proposed by popular health and beauty magazines may in fact be appropriate for a limited portion of the population. If you possess a mixed metabolic profile, then such "health and beauty tips" may work to a limited extent if your diet is appropriate for you. Even if you are biochemically mixed, but you are engaged in a dietary plan which is not appropriate for you, then all of the vitamins and minerals in the world will not do much to help you. If you are not biochemically mixed then following popular "health tips" results in a hit and miss type of strategy. This strategy may eventually backfire. You should now be aware that if two individuals possess similar symptoms they need not necessarily be identical biochemically. Hence the nutritional regimen appropriate for one individual may be completely inap-propriate for another.

Q: *How many biochemical types are there?*

A: Strictly speaking there is an infinite number of biochemical types. For the sake of simplicity I have divided the acid/alkaline spectrum into three arbitrarily designated categories, extremely acidic, mixed, and extremely alkaline. These categories must also be permuted over different periods of time. Hence if we take time variations into consideration, there are literally thousands of different biochemical types. Remember, some individuals oscillate over a 24 hour period while some oscillate over a period of approximately 28 days. Other individuals, and these cases are rare, oscillate both over 24 hours and within 28 days. Some individuals, and these cases are also rare, oscillate seasonally. Seasonal oscillation is the root cause of seasonal effective disorder or SAD. Occasionally individuals (and these cases are *extremely* rare), randomly jump from one point on the acid/alkaline scale to another within periods of hours.

Q: *Even though I've been told that I'm within normal limits by countless physicians thus far, wouldn't it be wise for me to visit just one more physician, one more time just to be sure I don't have a real medical problem?*

A: If you are asking this question I would suggest that you reread this book. You sound like one of many individuals suffering from what I call the *Marcus Welby Syndrome*. Marcus Welby, M.D. was the title of a popular television show in the 1960s. Friendly, venerable Dr. Welby, the show's protagonist, would invariably treat individuals who were by and large failed by the medical profession. They would come to Dr. Welby and describe their symptoms yet another time and Dr. Welby would lock on to a significant phrase in that description, pull out an obscure medical text, and immediately diagnose the patient's illness. This is the stuff of which fairy tales and Hollywood movies are made. This rarely happens in the real world. If you have been repeatedly failed by the medical profession, then chances are excellent that your problem is being caused by a substantial biochemical imbalance which lends itself to treatment via BioBalancing. If BioBalancing doesn't work let me assure you that the medical and psychiatric communities will be ready to receive you with open arms.

Q: *How can you say that biochemical problems are genetic? Speaking for myself, I have generally felt very well for a number of years and then suddenly my problem began without being caused by any identifiable external cause. If my problem is truly genetic, wouldn't I have been born with it and wouldn't it have been plaguing me for my entire life?*

A: Some genetic malfunctions manifest themselves in what I call "long trigger" or delayed fashion. It is therefore not unusual for example for a young girl to generally feel quite well up until the time she starts menstruating. At that time her acid/alkaline profile may start to undergo some very dramatic changes. These dramatic changes are by and large genetically programmed. Nevertheless I cannot emphasize too strongly that these genetic malfunctions can be countered nutritionally. Acid/alkaline nutrition will not alter your genetic structure, but it will counter-effect the manner in which your genetic problem is being expressed biochemically.

Q: *How can my problem be nutritional if I've always eaten the same way, but my problem only recently emerged?*

A: Within the context of BioBalance, if your nutritional regimen was not completely appropriate for your biochemical type, then your biochemistry probably underwent a slow but steady process of deterioration. Your problem will manifest itself when you have deteriorated beyond a maximum allowable limit.

The other possibility is that you have reached a significant biochemical "milestone" which I've already discussed earlier in this chapter.

Q: *If I prepare the meals in my household, what guarantee will I have that meals appropriate for me will be appropriate for everyone in my family?*

A: There is no guarantee. Ideally everyone in your household should know his or her metabolic/biochemical type and eat accordingly. As you can well imagine, if there are many people in your household, and if their biochemical types are substantially different, then preparing meals which are extremely varied can be difficult. It is helpful in a case like this to have supportive family members.

Q: *How long does it take to get into BioBalance?*

A: Approximately one individual in five is literally within a few meals of recovery. On the average however, it takes approximately 120 days to achieve BioBalance. Please note, I am not telling you that nothing happens by day 120 and then you are suddenly and miraculously brought into BioBalance on day 121. I'm saying that it is a process which occurs gradually over a three to four month period. Significant changes frequently occur within one to two weeks.

Q: *How long does it take to get rid of candidiasis?*

A: It generally takes approximately 90 days. A reliable method for getting rid of candidiasis is outlined in the next chapter.

Q: *If I have candidiasis and I get rid of it, can I then eat foods which were previously avoided as candida-inducing?*

A: Some people can and some people can't. I never suggest that anyone let his or her guard down completely insofar as candida is concerned. At this time I know of no biological indicator which can tell in advance if you are at high risk for contracting candidiasis after your candida levels have been brought under control.

Q: *What's the biggest shortcoming regarding BioBalancing?*

A: You generally have to stick to your regimen or set of regimens and keep diaries for a period of several months. This may sound easy, but I can assure you that it is hard work. If you are not willing to put in the effort, then chances are you're going to stay diseased. Typically, there is no "quick fix." If you don't want to make the effort, then BioBalancing is not for you.

Q: *But I feel I must eat whatever I want whenever I want it. What do I do to change my attitude?*

A: After you have deciphered your biochemical profile, I would suggest that you engage in a nutritional regimen appropriate for your biochemical *opposite*, in other words that you start eating only those foods which are inappropriate for you. You will rapidly deteriorate biochemically and likely experience some fairly substantial problems. The question you should ask yourself is the following, "Do I want to feel this way for the rest of my life?" You will ultimately wind up that way if you engage in indiscriminate eating practices.

Q: *Isn't BioBalancing just power of suggestion?*

A: If you are asking this question then you have missed the point I've been making in this book. Read my article published in the

International Journal of Biosocial Research (see references) to discover why so-called power of suggestion plays little if any role in BioBalance Therapy. An individual whose BioProfile changes in time will suddenly react adversely to a diet that agreed with him or her prior to the time when his or her biochemistry underwent a reversal. Power of suggestion cannot account for this.

Q: *Aren't you wrong in stating that each food has acid-inducing or alkaline-inducing properties. Don't the acid-inducing and alkaline-inducing properties of food depend upon the person eating them? In other words, while tomatoes for example may be acid-inducing for one individual they may be alkaline-inducing for another? Isn't that a more accurate account of what's going on here?*

A: Absolutely not. The acid/alkaline induction properties of foods are relatively independent of the individual ingesting them. There are some individual-specific variations, but they are insignificant. Some people who are philosophically predisposed to vegetarianism have a real problem understanding this point. They seem to be adamant about the belief that red meat is acid-inducing or becomes so after you have been a vegetarian long enough. That's simply not true. Remember, the acid/alkaline measure that is indicative of your overall status is venous plasma pH. Saliva pH, arterial pH, skin pH, urine pH, fecal pH, tear pH, toenail and fingernail pH, and hair pH among others are not always reliable.

Q: *But how can you attack psychotherapists? So many psychotherapists are such wonderful people.*

A: I am not attacking psychotherapists. I am attacking psychotherapy. I do not doubt for one moment that there are psychotherapists, possibly a great number of them who are indeed compassionate, well-meaning and well-intentioned people. Nonetheless I should point out that the road to hell is paved with good intentions. The real compassion of psychotherapists is yet to be put to the test. If they read and understand what it is that I am saying in this book, they will be faced with a decision, and that decision consists of continuing their practice and making more money or simply giving it up in order to better assist their patients. That's the real test. Sadly, I have already seen far too many "wonderful psychotherapists" who've made the wrong decision. I often wonder exactly how "wonderful" they can be to put their patients through such turmoil when there is an alternative.

Q: *But why can't you just keep an open mind and view psychotherapy as something that might be used in conjunction with BioBalancing?*

A: What's the sense of combining a mode of treatment which is more than 90% successful with a mode of treatment with a low success rate? I really have nothing against "talking things over" if the business of "talking things over" were deregulated and wouldn't cost you and me and society at large any additional financial hardships. My friends are the nicest people I know. I would much sooner "talk things over" with them at no cost to you, me and society in general in a time of social crisis, than spend large amounts of money talking to a qualified professional who hasn't the vaguest idea as to what makes me tick metabolically.

Keeping "an open mind" in terms of accepting the value of psychotherapy does not really constitute an intelligent decision at all in light of the evidence. In terms of dealing with the real world, I tell my friends that I can accept anything but a contradiction. If a statement is either self-contradictory or if its implications result in contradictions, then I will simply not accept that statement. I would wager further, that you wouldn't accept it either. There is a difference between being intellectually tolerant and being intellectually permissive. Tolerance implies accepting equivalent and viable alternatives. Permissiveness implies an "anything goes" philosophy, where the "anything" in question is not given the benefit of any scrutiny. Simply stated, if you stand for anything, you fall for everything. It's possible for an individual to have too open a mind. If you still persist and wonder why I'm not keeping "an open mind" in reference to psychotherapy then let me make the following remark in the context of the answer I have given you thus far: an open mind has but one disadvantage, it collects dirt.

Q: *Aren't you making grandiose claims for BioBalance Therapy by claiming that it's a cure-all?*

A: If you're asking this question then you've missed the point of this book. I suggest that you reread it. I've stated time and time again that

BioBalancing while revolutionary in its accomplishments and realm of application is not a panacea. The research I've conducted demonstrates this claim. Success was reported in gradients. It's not a matter of all or nothing.

Q: *You attack too many philosophies and therapies in complementary and alternative medicine (also known as holistic medicine). Some people get well as a result of techniques employed by holistic physicians without either the patient or the physician knowing why recovery occurred. This doesn't stop the physician from making grandiose claims about the technique that was used. But isn't that exactly what you're doing in this book with BioBalancing?*

A: I have not attacked holistic medicine in general. I am, however, rather unhappy with the turn of events that some holistic physicians have taken. Having spoken with numerous individuals who have spent a great deal of time and money under the care of holistic physicians I have observed that the following diagnoses seem to be widely prevalent at this time: weak adrenals, hypoglycemia, food/environmental allergies, candidiasis, deficient stomach acidity, pancreatitis, vitamin deficiency, more recently Epstein-Barr syndrome, and (of course, when all else fails) "stress." There is no doubt in my mind that some individuals are responsive to treatment for these disorders, but I am forced to conclude that only a minority respond favorably, and even a smaller minority respond to the many so-called "stress management" programs.

Yet it is noteworthy that these disorders have responded to BioBalance Therapy without any other complementary therapy. It's easy to jump to an erroneous conclusion, put words in my mouth and state that I am trying to convince you that in fact "BioBalancing is everything!." I never said that because it simply isn't true. I've been very careful to qualify virtually every claim I've made. In this regard I have made no such grandiose claims. Now, if you view BioBalancing as just another type of therapy that holistic physicians might use along with everything else, you will find in far too many cases (although certainly not all) that BioBalancing's 'tail' will soon wind up wagging holistic therapy's 'dog.'

Sadly, I have found talking to some holistic physicians a very frustrating experience. They are usually polite and intelligent, and never call BioBalancing quackery as many of their more orthodox counterparts have done. Their response typically goes as follows,

"Yeah sounds great, but I'm just too tied up right now." I will state again that I believe it would be irresponsible for holistic physicians to abandon all other modalities and therapies to, in essence, become 'BioBalance Therapists.' Nonetheless, when I hear holistic physicians tell me that one third to one half of their time is spent treating candida, I get frustrated.

On occasion, a holistic physician might elect to have a particular patient go through a program of BioBalance Therapy as a *test case*. Invariably, that patient will be what I call an "impossible case." The rationale the holistic physician employs argues that if the so-called impossible case gets well then BioBalancing can work miracles. This type of test is absolutely meaningless irrespective of the outcome. BioBalance Therapy cannot resurrect the dead. Priorities within the holistic health care community are going to have to change if holistic medicine is to right the wrongs made by medical orthodoxy and if holistic medicine is to become a real alternative and not just another trendy fad.

Q: *Now I for one am a believer in treating the whole person, you know, both mind and body. Isn't BioBalancing too lopsided in that regard?*

A: Me too. No, BioBalancing isn't lopsided at all.

Q: Are there any other books which discuss biochemical individuality in the same or similar fashion as this book?

A: Yes. Having spent the better part of twenty years researching the popular and scientific literature I can state that to my knowledge there are only two books, other than this one, published by the popular press which make an effort to scientifically validate the mechanism underlying the food-mood-health connection. These books are: *Nutrition and Your Mind: The Psychochemical Response* and *Personality Strength and Psychochemical Energy*, both authored by Dr. George Watson.

George Watson made an incalculable and indelible contribution to the field of psychonutrition and human health. He was probably the first serious researcher to formally recognize biochemical differences within any given population. In this context, he was also the first to realize that alterations in the rate at which you oxidize or burn up blood sugar are *intimately* connected to how you function psychologically. Dr. Watson discovered that dysfunctions in the mechanism underlying blood sugar metabolism and not "social factors" are primarily responsible for disorders commonly and erroneously classified as "psychological." The variable which Dr. Watson used to characterize individuals was intermediary metabolic oxidation rate, which incidentally correlates closely with acid/alkaline biochemistry. The major flaw I find in Watson's methodology lies with the tests that he developed to determine oxidative type, which he discusses in his books. After researching those tests extensively I have found that they do not provide an accurate indication of oxidative type and that they can be misleading in that regard. Nevertheless, Watson's contribution to the solution of the food-mood-health puzzle is enormous.

Q: *Are there any other naturally occurring factors other than food which may effect human health and behavior?*

A: Yes. For example, John Ott has spent the better part of his lifetime researching the impact of light upon human health. I cannot too strongly emphasize that to my knowledge, much of his work has not undergone the type of scrutiny I discuss here. Nevertheless I find Ott's observations very provocative. In this regard, I would speculate that BioBalancing's success rate could be substantially increased through the use of the techniques that Ott suggests. As I already stated, I have not received any funding for my own research, consequently I have exhausted my own funds and have had neither the time nor the money to test Ott's claims. If you are interested in learning more about John Ott's work on the effects of full spectrum radiation and health, I would suggest that you read his books *Light and Health, Light Radiation and You*, and, *Color and Light: Their Effects on Plants, Animals and People, Parts 1-5* (see references).

Q: *There are many foods which are not listed in the Appendix. How will I know if I should eat them?*

A: Good question. Simply achieve BioBalance using the methods outlined in the next chapter using *only* the foods listed in this book, and then introduce other foods (one at a time) to determine their effects. It's important to understand that a state of BioBalance is analogous to driving down a four lane super highway. If you steer clear of oncoming traffic and if you stay off the shoulder of the road you should do well. Being in BioBalance is *not* analogous to walking a tightrope where one false move will be fatal. Occasionally eating a *small* amount of food which should otherwise be avoided will not be disastrous. Nonetheless, I would urge you to be rigorous during the recovery phase and to remember that every person has a different margin of response to error or "cheating," so be careful.

Q: *With the exception of one brief anecdote, you haven't talked about the impact of BioBalancing upon nonhumans. For example, can BioBalance be used to improve the performance of race horses and racing dogs?*

A: An excellent question. I haven't addressed this topic because I haven't had the time or money to research it. I can however share some observations regarding my own pets. I have owned two large dogs and two cats. Three of the animals were alkaline and displayed remarkable improvement in their health and behavior after being placed on a quasi vegetarian diets with companion supplements. This incidentally seems to argue against a great deal of conventional wisdom regarding what is "naturally" good for dogs and cats in that they are generally viewed as being carnivorous in a "natural" state. The other animal (a dog) was slightly acidic and required a regimen rich in red meat and fish. All of the animals thrived. Because I do not jump to conclusions and make grandiose claims and sweeping generalizations, I won't try to convince you that these observations mean any more than what I report here. Nonetheless they are very suggestive and warrant additional research. If my suspicions are borne out, BioBalancing might impact veterinary medicine in much the same fashion that I hope it will impact other branches of medicine.

Q: I'm a health care practitioner and I'd like to incorporate BioBalance Therapy into my practice. How do I go about drawing blood and what type of plasmometer do I use.

A: Blood may be drawn from the antecubital vein. A regular 10 cc #20 syringe may be used. Approximately 5 cc of blood should suffice. The blood sample should be centrifuged for 2 to 3 minutes in a plain vacuum tube. A Clay-Adams CT-3300 SP centrifuge (or any equivalent model) is satisfactory. Venous plasma pH should be measured within 2 to 3 minutes after it is drawn, and therefore immediately after it has been centrifuged.

A plasmometer (Bench Top pH ATC Meter; Model SA 520; cat. no. 251-448052000) may be purchased from Orion Research, Inc. at 529 Main Street, Boston, MA 02129. Insofar as testing is concerned, you must follow the directions given in my book as explicitly as possible in order for your results to be meaningful. Also, you must be sure to calibrate your plasmometer as per the manufacturer's specifications so as to retain accuracy. You may use any plasmometer provided that it can accurately and reliably measure venous plasma pH to the one hundredths place.

In this regard, you should be suspicious of meter malfunction if pH values consistently rise above the low 7.50s or drop below the high 7.30s. Individuals possessing venous plasma pH values in these ranges are generally extremely distressed and psychotic (if symptoms manifest themselves in behavioral fashion).

IX

How To Determine Your BioProfile, Achieve BioBalance and Attain Peak Performance

---

WARNING

Despite the fact that you may have the constitutional right to self direct your own program of BioBalance Therapy, I feel legally compelled to tell you that you should only undergo BioBalance Therapy under the direct supervision of a licensed physician.

This chapter is divided into two "How To" sections. Section 1 explains how to undertake BioBalance Therapy using the results of blood analyses, while Section 2 will show you how to undertake BioBalance Therapy without blood tests. Section 2, unlike the first section outlines a trial and error approach.

SECTION 1.

You may initiate BioBalance Therapy by following these instructions:

1) Place yourself in one of the two following categories:

   A) any woman who is cycling menstrually; this category would include a woman who may have had a partial hysterectomy but

B) who has not undergone an öopherectomy and who claims to still have a "sense" of her cycle.

B) everyone else; if you are a woman and you are not certain as to whether you are ovulating or you have no apparent sense of your cycle then you would fall into this category as well.

Your physician must authorize a licensed laboratory to perform the tests which are discussed below. If your physician can find no such laboratory then he or she may purchase the equipment necessary to perform the blood tests on an inpatient basis by contacting a distributor of medical and scientific instruments.

If you fall into category "A" (above) you will undergo a series of blood tests for venous plasma pH (*not arterial pH*) and a test for candidiasis (antibody subclass IgG, IgA and IgM). *It is critical that venous plasma pH be measured to within one part in one hundred (two places to the right of the decimal) otherwise it will not be possible to determine your BioProfile.* While a series of blood draws will be required to determine variations in venous plasma pH, only one test for candidiasis need be performed. The test for candidiasis may be performed at any time.

Venous plasma pH will be measured at various times during each of three days. Each of these three days will correspond to one day in each of three respective phases of your menstrual cycle which are defined as follows: "premenstrual," in the *ideal* cycle refers to days 14 through 28; "menstrual," in the *ideal* cycle refers to days 1 through 4 or 5; "preovulatory," in the *ideal* cycle refers to days 5 through 14. Irrespective of the regularity of your cycle, you should be tested during any day within a two to five day period before the onset of menstruation, again during any day while you are menstruating, and again during any day within a two to five day period after menstruation has ended. Spotting at this time only is defined as menstruation.

During each of the three test days (each being representative of a different phase of the menstrual cycle) 4 blood samples will be drawn: 1) one sample before breakfast, 2) one sample midmorning, midway between breakfast and lunch, 3) one sample midafternoon, midway between lunch and dinner, and 4) one sample approximately two to three hours after dinner. Therefore, ideally 4 samples collected per day X 3 representative cycle phase-days equals 12 samples collected in total. If it is not possible to have blood drawn after dinner, then this sample may be excluded. However, for the sake of accuracy and completeness you should be encouraged to put up with the inconvenience, have an early dinner and have the fourth sample drawn approximately two to three hours after that meal.

For the sake of accurate record keeping, each sample should be appropriately identified as follows: name, date, time of day, phase of menstrual cycle (menstrual, preovulatory or premenstrual as defined above), and any one of the four following phrases: "before breakfast," "midway between breakfast and lunch," "midway between lunch and dinner," "after dinner."

PLEASE BE CERTAIN THAT THE FACILITY CONDUCTING THESE ANALYSES UNDERSTANDS THESE DIRECTIONS. TO REPEAT, IT IS CRITICAL THAT VENOUS PLASMA pH BE MEASURED TO THE NEAREST HUNDREDTH SUCH AS "7.41" or "7.46." DATA LISTED AS "7.4" IS NOT SIGNIFICANT.

If you fall into category "B," you may undergo the same test on any day as described above. Testing here is done in identical fashion as above, only now you will have four (4) blood samples drawn on the same day (before breakfast, between meals and evening).

Enclosed, at the end of this chapter, is a copy of a standardized food-mood diary form. For the sake of record keeping you should complete a copy of this form each day blood testing is performed. If you fall into category "A," you should designate the phase of your menstrual cycle in the upper right hand corner on each of 3 diary sheets that you will complete on each representative phase-day when you undergo blood testing. Despite the fact that challenge meals have been listed below, you should nevertheless fill in all of the information about food and moods. After the test day or between test days as the case may be, you may resume eating in any fashion. The following lists how you should eat on the day(s) of your blood tests.

Breakfast: 1 cup *regular* black coffee without sugar (*not* decaffeinated); 1 orange or tangerine, 1 rice cake (any variety, unsalted), one 8 ounce glass of water.

Mid Morning: 1 to 2 glasses of water (8 ounces each).

Lunch: Salad: Lettuce (any variety), tomatoes (any variety), onions (any variety including scallions), green pepper, shredded cabbage (any variety); dressing to consist of fresh squeezed lemon juice, 1 teaspoon of safflower or corn oil, and pressed garlic or fresh minced garlic; one to two glasses of water (8 ounces each), one 6 ounce cup of plain low fat yogurt. (You may wish to prepare this meal the night before the day of the blood test and place it in a sealable plastic bag).

Mid Afternoon: 1 to 2 glasses of water (8 ounces each).

Dinner: 4 ounces of chicken breast, baked or broiled (not fried) and skinned; 1 baked potato; broccoli (raw, steamed or boiled). One 8 ounce glass of water. (You may wish to prepare this meal the night before the day of the blood test and place it in a sealable plastic bag).

Mid Evening: 1 to 2 glasses of water (8 ounces each).

You may eat as much as you desire within reasonable limits where quantities are unspecified. You should not add any other condiments to these meals (ie., no salt, no butter, etc.). You may drink water at any time during the day without recording it in the diary. On the day(s) of the test, you should not have any snacks, vitamin/mineral supplements and if possible, no medications. You should abstain from medications pending your physician's approval. If you cannot suspend your medications, then you should list on the diary sheet(s) those medications which have been taken, the amount and the time when taken. If you are a smoker, you should list approximately how much tobacco has been smoked during the day(s) in question. You may do so by entering the approximate amount at the bottom of the diary sheet(s).

Mood descriptions should be brief and concise... "hyper," "agitated," "calm," "depressed," "relaxed," "poor concentration," "hostile," "panicky," etc. If you suffer physical symptoms as well, they should be listed along with moods... "headache," "sinus congestion," "backache," "nausea," etc. Since you will be drinking water at the specified "snack times on the test day(s), the phrase "1 (or 2 as the case may be) glass(es) of water" should be entered in the space next to the word "snack" on the diary. You must always record your moods and/or physical sensations if any, at all of the times indicated on the diary forms, even between meals despite the fact that no snacks will be eaten.

This is how you may analyze the results.

To avoid confusion it is worthwhile to review a key statement made earlier in this book. It was stated that in many cases BioBalance is achieved when venous plasma pH settles on a value in the immediate neighborhood of 7.46. It is critical to understand that each of the three steady state metabolic types discussed in this book achieve this value through *different* nutritional means. Since the standardized test meals listed above in this chapter are all *acid-inducing* and thus appropriate *only* for alkaline types, the following results are anticipated during the test day(s) when blood is drawn and venous plasma pH measured:

1. Acidic types will be forced into a state of substantial acidosis. Diurnal values of pH for most acidics will likely be below 7.46 and may drop substantially below 7.46 as the day progresses. Consequently, acidic types will generally report feeling worse than usual on the test day(s).

2. Mixed types will be forced into a state of significant and temporary acidosis. This state will usually not last for the entire day in that many mixed types are genetically programmed to rebound from the acidosis induced by the challenge meals later in the day. Diurnal values of pH for most mixed types will likely initiate at or below 7.46, drop below 7.46 as the day progresses and then climb back into the neighborhood 7.46 after dinner. Consequently, mixed types will generally report feeling worse than usual during much of the test day(s) with a period of remission in the early evening possibly extending into the late evening.

3. Alkaline types will be forced into a state of reduced alkalosis and possibly into a state of BioBalance. Diurnal values of pH for most alkaline types will initiate above 7.46 and either remain in the immediate neighborhood of the first measured early morning value, or drop to values in the neighborhood of 7.46 as the day progresses. Pre-existing symptoms may be expected to periodically break through during the day only to be lessened in intensity after each meal. Consequently, alkaline types will either generally report feeling the same as usual during much of the test day(s) or they will report a decrease/elimination of symptom severity.

Please keep in mind that BioBalance Therapy does not offer a miracle cure in that it generally takes approximately three months for an individual to derive full benefits from this program. Hence while some individuals may report substantial lessening of symptoms during one or more of the test days, many will not.

The following provides an actual example involving all three biochemical types. This BioProfile is that of a premenopausal woman. Once again, the downward trend in venous plasma pH is due to the extreme acid inducing nature of the challenge meals. During the mixed metabolic phase of this woman's cycle, she rebounded for the reasons given above.

Test Day	pH	Mood/Symptom Summary
Day #2 (menstrual phase):	early morning pH = 7.45	O.K.
	mid morning pH = 7.43	Nervous
	mid afternoon pH = 7.41	Nauseous/Panicky
(rebounding)...	mid evening pH = 7.45	Better
Day #7 (preovulatory phase):	early morning pH = 7.43	Very Tired
	mid morning pH = 7.41	Badly Depressed
	mid afternoon pH = 7.40	Crying
	mid evening pH = 7.41	Exhausted
Day #18 (premenstrual phase):	early morning pH = 7.49	Irritable
	mid morning pH = 7.47	Better
	mid afternoon pH = 7.46	Much Better
	mid evening pH = 7.47	O.K.

This woman is biochemically mixed during the menstrual phase, acidic during the preovulatory phase and alkaline during the premenstrual phase. The three nutritional regimens she will require to achieve BioBalance are given in the Appendix. Her nutritional regimens will vary depending upon the phase of her menstrual cycle.

There are some cases where the test days selected for cycling females are not representative of that woman's acid/alkaline cycle even though they may be representative of her menstrual cycle. For example, one woman was found to metabolize in a mixed mode throughout her entire cycle with the exception of the day of ovulation (when she became alkaline for 24 hours), and during a period starting 4 days before the onset of menstruation and ending on the second day of menstruation (during which she remained alkaline). *Admittedly, these cases are quite rare.* You should try to screen yourself for this eventuality so that you may schedule blood tests accordingly. When in doubt of course you may always schedule additional tests for venous plasma pH. Ideally you would want to obtain a pH trajectory on a daily basis, and seasonally in cases of seasonal affective disorder. This is clearly not feasible.

If your pH varies by more than 0.10 on any given day, you are probably a diurnal cycler. Your acid/alkaline imbalance cycles rhythmically on the day in question. Most diurnal cyclers start the day in an extreme alkaline state and end the day in an extreme acidic state. Here's an example of a diurnal cycler's pH over the course of one day:

Time	pH	State	Mood/Symptom Summary
early morning	pH = 7.50	extremely alkaline	*Very* Depressed
mid morning	pH = 7.48	mildly alkaline	Somewhat better
mid afternoon	pH = 7.44	mildly acidic	A little shakey
mid evening	pH = 7.39	extremely acidic	*Extremely* Agitated

If your venous plasma pH cycles in this manner then you should eat in a fashion appropriate for your biochemical state as given in the Appendix, *by varying your regimen depending upon the time of day.*

I cannot emphasize too strongly that there are always exceptions to these rules. Exceptions are to be expected in a field as complex as human biochemistry. There are some acidic individuals whose pH values are high. Similarly, there are some alkaline individuals whose pH values are low. Finally, there are some individuals whose pH values lie in the "normal" area who do not possess a mixed metabolic profile. These deviations can be accounted for through BioBalance Set Point Theory which I am currently attempting to develop. BioBalance Set Point Theory is far too complex to describe in this book, however it suffices to say that an attempt is being made to unravel these cases as well. Nonetheless, while BioBalance Therapy can be tailored for each individual, it is safe to say that the chances are good that you will fall into one or a combination of the three categories described here and that you can guide yourself through a program of BioBalance Therapy as indicated in the Appendix.

Irrespective of your biochemical type, *never* take any vitamin/mineral supplements *until* you are certain of your BioProfile. At least 30 days should be dedicated to adjusting your nutritional regimen(s) *before* you take any supplements (Appendix). If you react poorly to supplements, despite the fact that you are certain that these supplements are indeed biochemically appropriate for your biochemical type, YOU SHOULD STOP TAKING THEM IMMEDIATELY! Too many individuals mistakenly believe that adverse reactions to supplements form some type of "discharge reaction" or "healing crisis." This interpretation is without merit.

If you don't have candidiasis, and you respond well nutritionally, then don't attempt candida treatment despite the fact that pre-existing symptoms may have been so-called "classic" candida symptoms.

If candida levels are pathologically high and you respond well to specific nutritional regimen(s), then don't worry about lowering those levels. If this is the case then it turns out that you were not reactive to candida after all and that the candida was not contributing to your distress in the first place.

If on the other hand, candida levels are high and your response to BioBalancing is limited, then a course of medication for candidiasis should be administered. Treatment with a candicidal derived from the essential fatty acid called caprylic acid is often effective. Caprylic acid is not a prescription item. Most health food stores carry it. Typically, each tablet contains approximately 100 milligrams of caprylic acid. A regimen which is generally effective is listed below. Follow-up monitoring under the supervision of a physician is recommended in that you may suffer a Herxheimer reaction. In case you are candida reactive, you should *temporarily* (90 days) reduce or avoid your intake of yeast, wheat, canned goods, concentrates, mushrooms, fermented products, steroids, antibiotics and oral contraceptives (see asterisked items in each of the regimens outlined in the Appendix).

The following describes a typical course of treatment for candidiasis.

week number	number of milligrams of caprylic acid daily
1	100 after breakfast
2	100 after breakfast 100 after lunch
3 through 8	100 after each meal
9	100 after breakfast 100 after lunch
10 through 26	100 after breakfast

SECTION 2.

If you cannot test for venous plasma pH you will have to proceed by trial and error. Start out by assuming that you are alkaline and that you have candidiasis. Consequently, adhere to the more restrictive regimen appropriate for alkaline types which is listed in the Appendix (asterisked items are to be avoided).

A word of warning is in order at this point if you are a premeno-pausal woman. If your are a woman who is still having periods or if you have a "sense" of having a menstrual cycle, then it is critical that you begin this trial and error program during a certain time of the month. That time should be either immediately after the menstrual phase has ended (day # 5 or 6 in the ideal cycle) or immediately after ovulation (day #14 or #15 in the ideal cycle). I say this for the following reason. You will want to spend as much time as possible in the same phase of your menstrual cycle while undergoing any given trial regimen. In this fashion if you suffer an adverse reaction early during this trial and error program you will know that this adverse reaction resulted from your having selected the inappropriate regimen, and not from your having entered a new phase of your cycle. Let me give you an example. Let's say you first adhere to the regimen appropriate for alkaline types on day #27, and then on day #28 - #1 you suffer an adverse reaction. How will you know if you can attribute that adverse reaction to the fact that your initial nutritional selection was inappropriate or if your reaction was due to a rhythmic change from an alkaline state to a nonalkaline state when your period was about to start? The answer is that you won't! That's precisely why your starting this type of trial and error program just prior to when your cycle is about to phase change (around day 28 or around day 14) is *not* suggested. If you follow through with my advice and you suffer an adverse reaction, it will probably be distinct and it will occur *within* 3 days or even *within* one day after you have engaged in a regimen inappropriate for your acid/alkaline type.

Incidentally, the sample diaries at the end of this chapter were completed by a woman who undertook this program on a trial and error basis and whose acid/alkaline biochemistry shifted gears 3 times in the course of her menstrual cycle. Do not however automatically assume that just because you are premenopausal that your BioProfile must be cyclic. Be very rigorous with your nutritional regimen(s) through your first cycle, and be especially observant if you note any *substantial* deterioration around the time you phase change (again, day 28 - 1, day 4 - 5 and day 14 in the ideal cycle). Women who undertake this type of trial and error program find that it is an excellent learning experience in that in a rewarding sense, they become very *cycle aware*. Women who are cyclic biochemically can generally tell to *within one hour* when their acid/alkaline biochemical state is about to transition.

Let's assume that by selecting the regimen appropriate for alkaline types you have selected the regimen appropriate for your BioProfile. In this case one of two things will occur within the first 3 days of the trial. If you are indeed alkaline then you will either note some rapid improvement or no change. In either case, you should continue adhering to the regimen in question.

If you are not alkaline you will likely record rapid psychophysiological deterioration. If this is the case then switch to the regimen appropriate for acidics (see the Appendix). If your response to the regimen appropriate for acidics is favorable or neutral (no change) then you should continue adhering to that regimen. If your response to the regimen appropriate for acidics is favorable and then *rapidly* becomes unfavorable (within the same phase for women) then you very likely possesses a mixed metabolic profile and the regimen appropriate for acidics (which is very alkaline inducing) has made you too alkaline. In that event you should switch to the regimen appropriate for mixed types (the Appendix) and adhere to that regimen.

Let me review what I just said in simple tabular form. *This table only applies if you are initiating BioBalance Therapy through the use of trial and error and you choose the regimen appropriate for alkaline types as your first trial regimen.* The word "positive" means favorable. The word "negative" means unfavorable. The word "neutral" means the absence of any noticeable reaction, either positive or negative.

By the time you have self-administered a mixed-mode regimen, you will have exhausted all other options. For this reason, the mixed-mode regimen is *not* listed in the left hand column of this table. In the event however that you respond well to the mixed mode regimen for an extended period of time and then phase change (as would be the case with a cycling female), you should reinitiate the trial and error process by readministering the regimen appropriate for alkaline types.

I would urge you to take up to 30 days (or more if necessary) to be sure that the nutritional regimen or regimens you have selected is/are appropriate. If of course you are immediately aware of the fact that a regimen is causing unpleasant side effects you will want to switch as I have described above.

Regimen Appropriate for	Response	Action You Should Take
Alkalines Types	Positive or Neutral	Stay with this regimen
Alkaline Types	Negative	Switch to the regimen appropriate for acidics
Acidic Types	Positive or Neutral	Stay with this regimen
Acidic Types	Negative especially if preceded by a by a (very) brief positive reaction	Switch to the regimen appropriate for mixed types

Once again, *never* introduce vitamin and mineral supplements until well after the 30 day time limit has elapsed and you are fairly certain that you have in fact deciphered your acid/alkaline BioProfile. If your reaction to a regimen is favorable but your reaction to the complementary supplements is unfavorable, then STOP TAKING THE SUPPLEMENTS!

Finally, if your improvement at the end of this program leaves something to be desired, you may wish to undergo candida treatment as outlined above.

You *must* keep accurate food-mood diaries throughout the entire program of BioBalance Therapy. I have provided you with a real-life detailed diary at the end of this chapter. This should give you a good example of a relatively complex BioProfile. You should not be as sloppy with your regimens. *I must re-emphasize that there are shades of gray in between the various categories I have been using throughout this book, and fine tuning a biochemical type often can be rewarding.* Nonetheless, the information in this chapter and in the Appendix should provide you with an excellent start. You will note that with few exceptions the regimen appropriate for acidic types and the regimen appropriate for alkaline types are essentially mirror images of each other while the regimen appropriate for mixed types is essentially an admixture of the two biased a bit more heavily in favor of the regimen appropriate for acidic types. Eventually you should become well enough acquainted with these regimens to improvise your meals.

ABOUT WEIGHT CONTROL

I would discourage most individuals from counting calories for an extended period of time. You might find it beneficial to count calories for a few days to get a feel for how much you ought to be eating to devise a workable weight management program. Here is a rough rule of thumb you might use in deciding how much you ought to eat. I cannot too strongly emphasize that weight control is highly individual-specific and that the rules listed below are only meant to serve as generalizations. It has been my observation that variations of plus or minus 50% of the values given below have been found to apply over a broad range of population. Only personal trial and error will fine tune these differences. Once again, the guidelines given below only provide a rule of thumb.

Caloric Intake: Daily caloric intake required to maintain weight will approximately equal ideal weight (pounds) multiplied by 18. If you wish to alter your weight, a 500 calorie per day variation in this number will permit variation in weight by 1 pound per week.

Protein Intake: In the acidic and mixed cases, daily protein intake (ounces) required to maintain present weight will approximately equal ideal weight (pounds) divided by 15. In the alkaline case, divide ideal weight (pounds) by 20 to compute total daily protein intake (ounces). If you wish to alter your weight, then prorate this number by a ratio whose numerator equals the number of calories consumed daily and whose denominator equals the number of calories which would otherwise be consumed daily in the event you wanted to maintain your present weight. One ounce of lean meat, fish or poultry has the approximate protein equivalent of 2 to 4 ounces of dairy or 1 egg. NOTE THAT YOU CANNOT INDISCRIMINATELY SUBSTITUTE DAIRY AND EGGS FOR ANIMAL PROTEIN. ACIDIC AND MIXED TYPES MUST USE WHOLE DAIRY AND EGGS AS CONDIMENTS ONLY, WHILE ALKALINE TYPES MAY DISPLACE A SUBSTANTIAL AMOUNT OF ANIMAL PROTEIN WITH LOW FAT AND SKIM DAIRY AND SOME EGGS. SEE THE APPENDIX FOR ADDITIONAL DETAILS REGARDING PROTEIN SUBSTITUTION.

Fat Intake: In the acidic and mixed case, fat intake should approximately equal 20% of total caloric intake. In the alkaline case, fat intake should approximately equal 15% of total caloric intake. One tablespoon of oil contains 90 to 120 calories. One restaurant sized pat of butter or margarine contains 20 to 30 calories. Once again, different oils as well as butter and margarines are not interchangeable. Read the Appendix to determine which supplemental fat you should be using. Finally, keep in mind that about half of the fat you will be consuming is hidden fat in your food. Therefore the amount of added fat you will need will range from 10% to 7.5% depending upon whether you are mixed/acidic on the one hand or alkaline on the other respectively.

Carbohydrate Intake: The remainder of your caloric intake will consist of complex carbohydrates as found in vegetables, grains and (where appropriate) fruits.

Example 1: An alkaline female weighing 140 pounds wants to reduce her weight to to an ideal limit of 120 pounds. How must she structure her weight management program?

She must first self-administer the nutritional regimen appropriate for alkaline types described in the Appendix. Then she can configure her weight management program as follows:

If she had wanted to maintain her weight, her daily caloric intake would equal the following: 120x18 = 2160 calories. Since she wants to lose weight she might set a goal of losing 2 pounds per week, thus achieving her ideal weight in 10 weeks. To lose 2 pounds per week she would consume 1160 calories per day during the weight reduction phase and 2160 calories per day during the weight maintenance phase.

During the weight maintenance phase she would consume the following number of ounces of meat, fish or poultry protein daily (or caloric equivalent in eggs/low fat dairy): 120/20 = 6 ounces. Since she wishes to lose weight, she will daily be consuming only the following number of ounces during the weight reduction phase: 6x(1160/2160) = 3.22 ounces.

If she had wanted to maintain her weight she would add approximately 0.075x2160 = 162 calories of fat to her food daily, trying to delay that added fat intake until later in the day. Since she wishes to lose weight she will daily be consuming only the following number of calories of added fat during the weight reduction phase: 162x(1160/2160) = 87 calories. An example of how she might eat is listed in the Appendix.

Example 2: An acidic male weighing 140 pounds wants to increase his weight to an ideal limit of 160 pounds. How must he structure his weight management program?

He must first self-administer the nutritional regimen appropriate for acidic types described in the Appendix. Then he can configure his weight management program as follows:

If he had wanted to maintain his weight, his daily caloric intake would equal the following: 160x18 = 2880 calories. Since he wants to gain weight he might set a goal of gaining 2 pounds per week, thus achieving his ideal weight in 10 weeks. To gain 2 pounds per week he would consume 3880 calories per day during the weight augmentation phase and 2880 calories per day during the weight maintenance phase.

During the weight maintenance phase he would consume the following number of ounces of meat, fish or poultry protein daily: 160/15 = 10.66 ounces. Since he wishes to gain weight he will be consuming the following number of ounces of meat, fish or poultry protein daily during the weight augmentation phase: 10.66x (3880/2880) = 14.36 ounces. If he had wanted to maintain his weight he would add approximately 0.10x2880 = 280 calories of fat to his food daily, distributing that intake evenly throughout the day. Since he wishes to increase weight he will be consuming the following number of calories of added fat daily during the weight augmentation phase: 280x(3880/2880) = 377 calories. An example of how he might eat is listed in the Appendix.

The food-mood diaries which follow provide an example of how an individual (Phyllis R.) was able to decipher her BioProfile through trail and error in the fashion which has already been described in this chapter. In comparing the food-mood diaries with the information provided in the Appendix you'll note that Phyllis R.'s BioProfile is described as follows:

Phase of Menstrual Cycle	Acid/Alkaline Type
menstrual phase (days 1-4)	acidic
pre-ovulatory (days 5-12)	alkaline
day of ovulation (day 13)	acidic
premenstrual (days 14-24)	alkaline

Note the Phyllis R.'s cycle is not "ideal" but that the trial-and-error method I've outlined here served her well.

Name: Phyllis R.   Day of Week
Phase of Menstrual Cycle: Premenstrual Day 18
Quality and duration of sleep - *71/2 hours - poor*
Time of awakening - *6:30 am*
Mood upon awakening - *tired, achy, depressed*

Time of Breakfast - *7:00 am*
Mood before Breakfast - *same*
Mood after Breakfast - *better, by no means 100%*
Breakfast - *coffee (regular) black, 1/2 grapefruit, 4 oz. yogurt*

Time of midmorning snack - *10:30 am*
Mood before snack - *hungry, tired (again)*
Mood after Snack - *alert, less achy*
Snack - *1 tangerine, 1 rice cake, 1 coffee (reg)*

Time of Lunch - *12:15 pm*
Mood before Lunch - *hungry, otherwise ok*
Mood after Lunch - *good*
Lunch - *chef's salad: lean ham, 1 egg, lettuce, tomato, cabbage, scallion, tea*

Time of midafternoon snack - *2:30 pm*
Mood before snack - *good*
Mood after snack - *good*
Snack - *none*

Time of Dinner - *6:30 pm*
Mood before Dinner - *a bit hungry, getting tired*
Mood after Dinner - *full, not as tired*
Dinner - *chicken breast in tomato sauce (lean), broccoli, brown rice, tea*

Time of afterdinner snack - *8:30 pm*
Mood before snack - *getting tired*
Mood after snack - *getting tired*
Snack - *none*

Time of retiring - *10:00 pm - asleep by 11:00 pm*
Mood upon retiring - *exhausted*

Morning exercise - *none*
Afternoon exercise - *none*
Evening exercise - *none*
(Describe duration of exercise and type as well as pulse where applicable.)

Name: Phyllis R.   Day of Week
Phase of Menstrual Cycle: Premenstrual day 19

Quality and duration of sleep - *71/2 - poor*
Time of awakening - *6:30 am*
Mood upon awakening - *lousy*

Time of Breakfast - *7:00 am*
Mood before Breakfast - *lousy*
Mood after Breakfast - *ok*
Breakfast - *1 coffee, 1 bowl corn flakes (sugar free), 1% milk, orange juice*

Time of midmorning snack - *10:30 am*
Mood before snack - *ok*
Mood after Snack - *pretty good*
Snack - *1 coffee & doughnut "hole" (a "no-no")*

Time of Lunch - *12:00 pm*
Mood before Lunch - *still good, getting hungry*
Mood after Lunch - *good*
Lunch - *tuna salad sandwich (white tuna, onions, mayo), pita bread, tea*

Time of midafternoon snack - *2:45*
Mood before snack - *getting tired*
Mood after snack - *waking up*
Snack - *coffee & doughnut "hole" (a "no-no")*

Time of Dinner - *6:45 pm*
Mood before Dinner - *pretty good*
Mood after Dinner - *good*
Dinner - *scrod, baked potato, 1 pat margarine, broccoli, 1 tspn sherbet*

Time of afterdinner snack - *9:00 pm*
Mood before snack - *not bad*
Mood after snack - *same*
Snack - *2 rice cakes toasted*

Time of retiring - *10:15 pm asleep by 11:00 pm*
Mood upon retiring - *tired (not exhausted)*

Morning exercise - *none*
Afternoon exercise - *took brisk 20 minute walk*
Evening exercise - *15 minutes rebound trampoline - 140 beats per minute*
(Describe duration of exercise and type as well as pulse where applicable.)

Name: Phyllis R.   Day of Week
Phase of Menstrual Cycle: Premenstrual day 20

Quality and duration of sleep - *71/2 - so-so, better than usual for time of cycle*
Time of awakening - *6:30*
Mood upon awakening - *half way human*

Time of Breakfast - *7:00 am*
Mood before Breakfast - *still not bad, a bit hungry*
Mood after Breakfast - *ok*
Breakfast - *1 soft boiled egg, 2 oz yogurt (lowfat), 1 coffee, essene bread*

Time of midmorning snack - *10:15*
Mood before snack - *just ok (barely), a little achy-lower back*
Mood after Snack - *much improved - almost no back ache*
Snack - *coffee & 1 apple*

Time of Lunch - *12:00 pm*
Mood before Lunch - *still good*
Mood after Lunch - *still good*
Lunch - *tuna salad sandwich with pita bread (see day #19) - boring*

Time of midafternoon snack - *2:34*
Mood before snack - *ok*
Mood after snack - *better*
Snack - *coffee & peach*

Time of Dinner - *8:00 pm (exercised 1st)*
Mood before Dinner - *GREAT!*
Mood after Dinner - *STILL GREAT!*
Dinner - *boiled ham, baked potato, steamed cabbage, 1 beer (lite)*

Time of afterdinner snack - *9:30*
Mood before snack - *good*
Mood after snack - *good*
Snack - *1 rice cake*

Time of retiring - *11:00 pm*
Mood upon retiring - *ok*

Morning exercise - *none*
Afternoon exercise - *brisk walk (20 minutes)*
Evening exercise - *1/2 hour aerobics at spa - 160 bpm*
(Describe duration of exercise and type as well as pulse where applicable.)

Name: Phyllis R.   Day of Week
Phase of Menstrual Cycle: Premenstrual day 21

Quality and duration of sleep - *71/2 hours - restful*
Time of awakening - *6:30*
Mood upon awakening - *not bad*

Time of Breakfast - *7:00 am*
Mood before Breakfast - *still not bad*
Mood after Breakfast - *good*
Breakfast - *bowl oatmeal & 1% milk, coffee, 1 melon wedge*

Time of midmorning snack - *10:45*
Mood before snack - *good*
Mood after Snack - *good*
Snack - *1 oatmeal cookie 1 coffee*

Time of Lunch - *12:15*
Mood before Lunch - *very good, energetic, cheerful*
Mood after Lunch - *still excellent*
Lunch - *roast beef, mashed potatoes & gravy, green beans, clam chowder*

Time of midafternoon snack - *2:30 pm*
Mood before snack - *very tired, somewhat depressed (must have been lunch)*
Mood after snack - *so-so*
Snack - *coffee*

Time of Dinner - *7:30*
Mood before Dinner - *Yuk!*
Mood after Dinner - *so-so no great shakes*
Dinner - *lean pork chop, zucchini, stewed tomatoes, chicken/barley broth*

Time of afterdinner snack -
Mood before snack - *tired*
Mood after snack - *tired*
Snack - none

Time of retiring - *9:30 pm - this is how exhausted I am!*
Mood upon retiring - *exhausted*

Morning exercise - *none*
Afternoon exercise - *none*
Evening exercise - *none*
(Describe duration of exercise and type as well as pulse where applicable.)

Name: Phyllis R.   Day of Week
Phase of Menstrual Cycle: Premenstrual day 22

Quality and duration of sleep - *9 1/2 hours - as though I were drugged*
Time of awakening - *7:00 am*
Mood upon awakening - *zombie - awful!*

Time of Breakfast - *n/a*
Mood before Breakfast - *same*
Mood after Breakfast - *a little better*
Breakfast - coffee - *no time had to leave (thank God it's Friday)*

Time of midmorning snack - *n/a - rushed - no time (10:30 am)*
Mood before snack - *surprisingly good*
Mood after Snack -
Snack -

Time of Lunch - n/a - *rushed had to meet deadline*
Mood before Lunch - *surprisingly good*
Mood after Lunch - *very good*
Lunch -

Time of midafternoon snack - *3:15 pm*
Mood before snack - *very good, rushed at work but calm*
Mood after snack - *energetic*
Snack - *1 coffee, thin slice rum cake ("no-no"), office party*

Time of Dinner - *8:30 pm (restaurant with boyfriend)*
Mood before Dinner - *great, up-beat, good sense of humor*
Mood after Dinner - *still excellent*
Dinner - *stuffed flounder (breaded) zucchini, wildrice, 1 bloody mary*

Time of afterdinner snack - *11:00 pm*
Mood before snack - *great*
Mood after snack - *winding down*
Snack - *none*

Time of retiring - *2:30 am*
Mood upon retiring - *tired but peaceful*

Morning exercise - *none*
Afternoon exercise - *brisk 20 minute walk*
Evening exercise - *1/2 hour rebound on trampoline 140 bpm*
(Describe duration of exercise and type as well as pulse where applicable.)

Name: Phyllis R.   Day of Week
Phase of Menstrual Cycle: Premenstrual day 23

Quality and duration of sleep - *8-1/2 hours*
Time of awakening - *11:00 am*
Mood upon awakening - *not bad considering period's due & went to bed late*

Time of brunch - *12:00 pm*
Mood before Breakfast -
Mood after Breakfast - *good*
Breakfast - *omelet (onions, pepper, tomatoes), essence bread, coffee*

Time of midafternoon snack - *3:00 pm*
Mood before snack - *good*
Mood after Snack - *none*
Snack - *good*

Time of Lunch -
Mood before Lunch -
Mood after Lunch - *good*
Lunch -

Time of midafternoon snack -
Mood before snack -
Mood after snack - *good*
Snack -

Time of Dinner - *7: pm*
Mood before Dinner - *a bit tired*
Mood after Dinner - *good*
Dinner - *salad ("allowed" veggies), turkey, tomato, brown rice, brussel sprouts*

Time of afterdinner snack -
Mood before snack -
Mood after snack -
Snack - *none*

Time of retiring - 1:00 am - *late night movie*
Mood upon retiring - *tired, hungry*

Morning exercise - *none*
Afternoon exercise - *1/2 hour aerobics 165 bpm*
Evening exercise - *20 minutes rebound trampoline 140 bpm*
(Describe duration of exercise and type as well as pulse where applicable.)

Name: Phyllis R.   Day of Week
Phase of Menstrual Cycle: Premenstrual day 24 — Menstrual day 1

Quality and duration of sleep - *7 hours*
Time of awakening - *8:00 am*
Mood upon awakening - *shakey, spacey, cramps*

Time of Breakfast - *rushed, went to church 8:45 am*
Mood before Breakfast - *shakey still*
Mood after Breakfast - *ok - very hungry*
Breakfast - *coffee & 1 slice essence bread*

Time of midmorning snack - *9:00 am*
Mood before snack - *very shakey, weepy*
Mood after Snack - *went home had a good cry (sermon? period?) - a bit better*
Snack - *none*

Time of Lunch - *1:00 pm*
Mood before Lunch - *shakey, nervous*
Mood after Lunch - *ok for 1/2 hour then awful, very tense, hyperventilating*
Lunch - *Bar B Q chicken breast, potato salad, raw broccoli*

Time of midafternoon snack - *2:15 pm*
Mood before snack - *awful*
Mood after snack - *extremely anxious, panicky! took 2 aspirins - not better*
Snack - *coffee to see if it helps) & orange*

Time of Dinner - *6:00 pm*
Mood before Dinner - *horrible, hot flashes, bad headache, anxious*
Mood after Dinner - *better but not 100%*
Dinner - *hamburger (6oz) potatoes fried in grease (ugh!), (frozen) spinach*

Time of afterdinner snack - *9:15 pm*
Mood before snack - *so-so, kind of hungry*
Mood after snack - *lots better*
Snack - *buttered popcorn & salt*

Time of retiring - *10:30 pm*
Mood upon retiring - *exhausted – perhaps I'm becoming acidic - try switching diet*

Morning exercise - *none*
Afternoon exercise - *none*
Evening exercise- *none*
(Describe duration of exercise and type as well as pulse where applicable.)

Name: Phyllis R.   Day of Week
Phase of Menstrual Cycle: Menstrual day 2

Quality and duration of sleep - *Sound - 7 hours - 5:30 am - earl;y for me*
Time of awakening - *5:30 am*
Mood upon awakening - *famished*

Time of Breakfast - *6:00 am*
Mood before Breakfast - *famished*
Mood after Breakfast - *good, energized*
Breakfast - *sausage patty & 1 fried egg in fat, essene bread, butter, decaf coffee*

Time of midmorning snack - *9:45 am*
Mood before snack - *good, but hungry, a bit jittery*
Mood after Snack - *better - full*
Snack - *1/2 avocado & raw cauliflower*

Time of Lunch - *12:00 pm*
Mood before Lunch - *good but hungry, somewhat jittery*
Mood after Lunch - *fine!*
Lunch - *beef stew & creamed spinach & fried cauliflower*

Time of midafternoon snack - *2:20 pm*
Mood before snack - *ok*
Mood after snack - *ok*
Snack - *1 decaf coffee & cream & handful of peanuts*

Time of Dinner - *6:30 pm*
Mood before Dinner - *hungry again!*
Mood after Dinner - *much better, full some energy*
Dinner - *salmon & cup of split pea soup & asparagus*

Time of afterdinner snack - *9:00 pm*
Mood before snack - *ok*
Mood after snack - *calm, relaxed*
Snack - *buttered popcorn & salt*

Time of retiring - *11:00 pm*
Mood upon retiring - *good, tired*

Morning exercise - *none*
Afternoon exercise - *none*
Evening exercise - *none*
(Describe duration of exercise and type as well as pulse where applicable.)

Name: Phyllis R.   Day of Week
Phase of Menstrual Cycle: Menstrual day 3

Quality and duration of sleep - sound - *9 hours*
Time of awakening - *6:00 am*
Mood upon awakening - *tired hungry*

Time of Breakfast - *6:30 am*
Mood before Breakfast - *tired, hungry*
Mood after Breakfast - *much better*
Breakfast - *hash browns, burger, weak tea & cream*

Time of midmorning snack - *10:30 am*
Mood before snack - *ok*
Mood after Snack - *ok*
Snack - none - *RUSHED*

Time of Lunch - *12:00 pm*
Mood before Lunch - *a bit shakey, nauseous*
Mood after Lunch - *funny*
Lunch - *chopped sirloin & NE clam chowder (no msg)*

Time of midafternoon snack - *2:15 pm*
Mood before snack - *good*
Mood after snack - *good, calm, energetic*
Snack - *carrot & rice cake with peanut butter*

Time of Dinner - *7:30 (worked out first)*
Mood before Dinner - *excellent*
Mood after Dinner - *excellent - still*
Dinner - *liver pate; (home made), brown rice with cream sauce*

Time of afterdinner snack - *8:45 pm*
Mood before snack - *winding down*
Mood after snack - *winding down*
Snack - *rice cake with butter*

Time of retiring - *11:30 (depressing 11:00 news)*
Mood upon retiring - *good - tired*

Morning exercise - *trampoline/rebound 20 minutes 140 bpm*
Afternoon exercise - *10 minute walk - brisk*
Evening exercise - *1/2 hour aerobics & free weights 160 bpm*
(Describe duration of exercise and type as well as pulse where applicable.)

Name: Phyllis R.   Day of Week
Phase of Menstrual Cycle: Menstrual day 4

Quality and duration of sleep - *7 hours - peaceful (1 erotic dream)*
Time of awakening - *6:30 am*
Mood upon awakening - *FINE*

Time of Breakfast - *7:00 am*
Mood before Breakfast - *fine*
Mood after Breakfast - *excellent*
Breakfast - *lamb patty, 1 fried egg, 1 cup of oats & cream*

Time of midmorning snack - *10:30 am*
Mood before snack - *good*
Mood after Snack - *good*
Snack - *decaf coffee & cream, 1 rice cake & peanut butter*

Time of Lunch - *12:15 pm*
Mood before Lunch - *good*
Mood after Lunch - *excellent!*
Lunch - *spare ribs, corn on the cob, lima beans*

Time of midafternoon snack - *3:00 pm*
Mood before snack - *good*
Mood after snack - *good*
Snack - *none*

Time of Dinner - *7:45 pm*
Mood before Dinner - *good*
Mood after Dinner - *fine*
Dinner - *tuna salad (dark tuna), 1 steamed artichoke, millet & butter*

Time of afterdinner snack - *9:45 pm*
Mood before snack - *ok*
Mood after snack - *ok*
Snack - *2 glasses water*

Time of retiring - *10:30 pm*
Mood upon retiring - *tired - thirsty*

Morning exercise - *20 minutes rebound/trampoline 140 bpm*
Afternoon exercise - *15 minutes brisk walk*
Evening exercise - *aerobics 165 bpm & free weights*
(Describe duration of exercise and type as well as pulse where applicable.)

Name: Phyllis R.   Day of Week
Phase of Menstrual Cycle: Preovulatory day 5

Quality and duration of sleep - *11 hours - awful*
Time of awakening - *8:45 am*
Mood upon awakening - *horrible, headache, backache, will be late for work*

Time of Breakfast - *9:00 am*
Mood before Breakfast - *awful*
Mood after Breakfast - *worse - phoned office - will be out sick*
Breakfast - *1 sausage link, essene bread & pat butter*

Time of midmorning snack - *none - diarrhea at 10:00 am*
Mood before snack - *throbbing headache*
Mood after Snack - *not much better*
Snack - weak tea

Time of Lunch - none -
Mood before Lunch - *sipped some tea - felt a bit better*
Mood after Lunch - *feel awful but not flu symptoms**
Lunch -

Time of midafternoon snack - *None*
Mood before snack -
Mood after snack -
Snack -

Time of Dinner - *8:30 pm*
Mood before Dinner - *tired & drawn*
Mood after Dinner - *poor but better than I've felt all day*
Dinner - *brown rice, 1 oz sole & lemon & tea*

Time of afterdinner snack - *none*
Mood before snack -
Mood after snack -
Snack -

Time of retiring - *9:30 pm*
Mood upon retiring - *beat – Perhaps I'm becoming alkaline again - try switching diet*

Morning exercise -
Afternoon exercise -
Evening exercise -
(Describe duration of exercise and type as well as pulse where applicable.)

Name: Phyllis R.   Day of Week
Phase of Menstrual Cycle: Preovulatory day 6

Quality and duration of sleep - *9 hours, good*
Time of awakening - *6:30*
Mood upon awakening - *much better - normal bowel movement*

Time of Breakfast - *7:00 am*
Mood before Breakfast - *ok*
Mood after Breakfast - *good, more energy*
Breakfast - *teas, lemon & 1 rice cake & 1 small bowl of cream of rice w/ honey*

Time of midmorning snack - *10:15 am*
Mood before snack - *good*
Mood after Snack - *good*
Snack -

Time of Lunch - *12:30 pm*
Mood before Lunch - *hungry, otherwise good*
Mood after Lunch - *good*
Lunch - *salad (allowed veggies) & lean ham (very little), tea*

Time of midafternoon snack - *rushed no time*
Mood before snack - *good mood, energetic*
Mood after snack -
Snack -

Time of Dinner - *8:30 pm*
Mood before Dinner - *GREAT!*
Mood after Dinner - *very good*
Dinner - *cod steak, baked potato, buckwheat, (no bad - eh?), cabbage*

Time of afterdinner snack - *none*
Mood before snack - *feeling fine*
Mood after snack -
Snack -

Time of retiring - *11:30*
Mood upon retiring - *tired but peaceful*

Morning exercise - *none*
Afternoon exercise - *20 minute walk, brisk*
Evening exercise - *1/2 hour aerobics & free weights*
(Describe duration of exercise and type as well as pulse where applicable.)

Name: Phyllis R.   Day of Week
Phase of Menstrual Cycle:

Quality and duration of sleep -
Time of awakening -
Mood upon awakening -

Time of Breakfast -
Mood before Breakfast -
Mood after Breakfast -
Breakfast -

Time of midmorning snack -   From day # 7 through day #12,
Mood before snack -   Phyllis reported repeatedly feeling
Mood after Snack -   well while remaining on the diet
Snack -   appropriate for alkaline types

Time of Lunch -
Mood before Lunch -
Mood after Lunch -
Lunch -

Time of midafternoon snack -
Mood before snack -
Mood after snack -
Snack -

Time of Dinner -
Mood before Dinner -
Mood after Dinner -
Dinner -

Time of afterdinner snack -
Mood before snack -
Mood after snack -
Snack -

Time of retiring -
Mood upon retiring -

Morning exercise -
Afternoon exercise -
Evening exercise -
(Describe duration of exercise and type as well as pulse where applicable.)

Name: Phyllis R.   Day of Week
Phase of Menstrual Cycle: Probably Ovulating Day 13

Quality and duration of sleep - *7 hours, good*
Time of awakening - *6:30 am*
Mood upon awakening - *good*

Time of Breakfast - *7:00 am*
Mood before Breakfast - *ok*
Mood after Breakfast - *ok then 1 hour later shakey*
Breakfast - *1 bowl wheatena & 1% milk, coffee, 1 glass orange juice*

Time of midmorning snack - *10:00 am*
Mood before snack - *very shakey*
Mood after Snack - *panic! very anxious, don't want to be in office -took valium***
Snack - *coffee & doughnut hole*

Time of Lunch - *12:00 pm*
Mood before Lunch - *dopey*
Mood after Lunch - *same*
Lunch - *none*

Time of midafternoon snack - *2:30 pm*
Mood before snack - *ok*
Mood after snack - *ok*
Snack - *decaf coffee with cream*

Time of Dinner - *7:00 pm*
Mood before Dinner - *ok*
Mood after Dinner - *better, not 100% but best I've felt all day*
Dinner - *sauteed chicken livers with bacon, steamed peas & carrots*

Time of afterdinner snack - *9:00 pm*
Mood before snack - *good*
Mood after snack - *good*
Snack - *popcorn & butter & salt*

Time of retiring - *9:45 pm -wish there were an easier way - I know there's none*
Mood upon retiring - *next time I'll be reincarnated as a man!!! Must be acidic on day of ovulation in mid cycle - watch out for day #13*

Morning exercise - *none*
Afternoon exercise - *none*
Evening exercise - *5 minutes rebound/trampoline 110 bpm*
(Describe duration of exercise and type as well as pulse where applicable.)

Name   Day of Week
Phase of Menstrual Cycle (Circle one)
                              Menstrual Premenstrual Preovulatory Other
Quality and duration of sleep -
Time of awakening -
Mood upon awakening -

Time of Breakfast -
Mood before Breakfast -
Mood after Breakfast -
Breakfast -

Time of midmorning snack -
Mood before snack -
Mood after Snack -
Snack -

Time of Lunch -
Mood before Lunch -
Mood after Lunch -
Lunch -

Time of midafternoon snack -
Mood before snack -
Mood after snack -
Snack -

Time of Dinner -
Mood before Dinner -
Mood after Dinner -
Dinner -

Time of afterdinner snack -
Mood before snack -
Mood after snack -
Snack -

Time of retiring -
Mood upon retiring -

Morning exercise -
Afternoon exercise -
Evening exercise -
(Describe duration of exercise and type as well as pulse where applicable.)

Name   Day of Week
Phase of Menstrual Cycle (Circle one)
                              Menstrual Premenstrual Preovulatory Other
Quality and duration of sleep -
Time of awakening -
Mood upon awakening -

Time of Breakfast -
Mood before Breakfast -
Mood after Breakfast -
Breakfast -

Time of midmorning snack -
Mood before snack -
Mood after Snack -
Snack -

Time of Lunch -
Mood before Lunch -
Mood after Lunch -
Lunch -

Time of midafternoon snack -
Mood before snack -
Mood after snack -
Snack -

Time of Dinner -
Mood before Dinner -
Mood after Dinner -
Dinner -

Time of afterdinner snack -
Mood before snack -
Mood after snack -
Snack -

Time of retiring -
Mood upon retiring -

Morning exercise -
Afternoon exercise -
Evening exercise -
(Describe duration of exercise and type as well as pulse where applicable.)

X

Conclusion:
Whom Do I Believe?

It is not uncommon for someone who has listened to me speak, to tell me that everything I said was interesting and that I seem like a bright and congenial person, but why should they believe me as opposed to anyone else? After having read most of my book you may feel the same way. After all, while my credentials may be impressive, so are the credentials of most other people writing books about nutrition. Some people ingenuously go so far as to tell me that if they had to decide on a diet, they would probably opt for a diet endorsed by a "real doctor" (namely a physician) as opposed to *my diet* since I only have a doctorate in physics. Some people after hearing me lecture throw their hands up in desperation and admit to being totally and completely confused. "The Feingold Diet, the Pritikin Diet, the Berger Diet, the Atkins Diet, the Randolph Diet, the Crook Diet, the Truss Diet, Macrobiotics, the Haas Diet. Whom do I believe?" they exclaim!

The question of *whom* you should believe is really a non-question. More appropriately stated the question should be, *"What* do I believe?"

Having been trained as a physicist, I am often amused when I see people in the social sciences, especially psychology, quoting established authorities. I always approach *experts* with some degree of suspicion. It is common practice in physics to ask someone lecturing in an area of physics to prove a specific statement or remark. If Albert Einstein were alive today and gave a seminar on general relativity and made a statement which was not apparently well-founded, I would be within my rights as a scientist to ask him to prove that remark. Proof could independently come in one of two forms: (1) Einstein could mathematically show me that the statement in question results logically from first or basic principles in physics which have been repeatedly shown to be correct, or (2) Einstein could tell me that while he cannot offhand see a connection between his statement and first principles of physics, he can show me that his statement can be experimentally verified.

The first method is called *deduction*, and the second is called *induction*. I would be foolish to run out of the lecture hall after hearing Einstein speak, quoting Einstein because, "Einstein said so!," only to find out later that Einstein was wrong. People who often want to be intellectually associated with Einstein will quote him on politics, religion and virtually anything. Einstein made numerous statements not pertaining to physics or science in general, many of which are contradictory. Ideally, in the scientific community credentials don't count for much when the chips are down. When you make a statement, any statement, you may and should be taken to task and asked to back that statement up.

A true scientist will not be embarrassed by having to back up or prove a statement. Shouting, theatrics, intimidation, *pointing to credentials*, or telling you to "trust me," don't carry much weight in legitimate scientific circles. A story has it that Albert Einstein was once lecturing a group of graduate students when one of the students asked him to prove a statement he had just made. Einstein replied that it was obvious, paced back and forth, left the classroom in deep thought and then returned half an hour later with a smile on his face reaffirming the fact that it was indeed obvious. He then went on to state his proof. Everyone was satisfied. There is a certain inner satisfaction, some have even called it a "high," that a physicist or mathematician feels when he or she can prove a statement relating to natural phenomena. Something "clicks" when you know you're right. When asked how he had come up with the theory of relativity, Einstein stated that whereas prior to this theory, all of his colleagues considered physics to be obvious and intuitive, he felt that physics was not obvious and intuitive, and indeed probably wrong! The idea you see, is to keep questioning until you come up with a contradiction or until you can prove what it is you are seeking to prove or disprove in terms of principles which have been verified time and time and time again.

How does all this apply to diet and psychology and medicine in general, you might ask? Oftentimes people (even well-educated people) tell me that while the laws of physics apply to electrons and stars, they don't apply to people. After all, I'm told, the behavior of people obeys the laws of *"psychologic"* and not the laws of logic or physics or any other well defined system of thought. Well, behavior does and it doesn't, but a detailed philosophical discussion of this point lies well beyond the scope of this book.

If you have understood what I have said thus far in this chapter, you might really despair and tell me, "You've got to be kidding! Do you mean I've got to become an expert in cardiology before I see my cardiologist; an expert in psychiatry before I see my psychiatrist; an expert in nutrition before I see my nutritionist; an expert in pharmacology before I talk to my druggist... all so that I can make sure that what these people will tell me is true or correct! Surely, trust enters somewhere into the equation, because if it doesn't I won't have enough time in my life to keep tabs on all these disciplines."

Well, you're right, and you're also wrong. Recall what I just said. There are two ways you can prove or disprove something, *deductively* and *inductively*. The first is difficult and time consuming. The second is easy and can be done in less than one minute. I'll show you how.

> *Once upon a time there was a young man who walked through the streets of London sprinkling powder wherever he walked. An old man walked up to him and asked, "What are you doing?" The young man answered, "Why I'm sprinkling Dr. Smith's Lion Powder, of course." The old man looked puzzled, "Lion Powder, what's that?" The young man smiled, "It keeps the lions off the streets of London." The old man burst out in laughter, "You silly young fool, don't you know that there are no lions on the streets of London!." The young man said triumphantly, "Of course there aren't! This powder really works!."*

You may think the young man was incredibly stupid or to be charitable, naive. Well, you'd be surprised at how many people approach numerous issues in the same fashion as the young man in this story. The most obvious criticism of the young man would be if he had stopped sprinkling the powder he would have realized that no lions prowled the streets of London without it. The continued absence of lions even after the application of the powder had ceased should have led the young man to conclude that Dr. Smith's powder was worthless. What questions should the young man have asked Dr. Smith before buying his powder and sprinkling it along the streets of London? I list them below.

1. What percentage of the population will report seeing lions if I sprinkle the powder?

2. What percentage of the population will report *not* seeing lions if I sprinkle the powder?

3. What percentage of the population will report seeing lions if I *don't* sprinkle the powder?

4. What percentage of the population will report *not* seeing lions if I *don't* sprinkle the powder?

Since a picture is worth a thousand words, I've put these questions in matrix or tabular form in Table 10:1.

	% of individuals observing lions	% of individuals *not* observing lions
with Dr. Smith's Lion Powder		
without Dr. Smith's Lion Powder		

Table 10:1.   The form that a table or matrix might take in determining the validity of the statement, "Dr. Smith's Lion Powder is effective in keeping Lions off the streets of London."

If prior to buying Dr. Smith's powder, the young man had presented Dr. Smith with the matrix given above and had asked Dr. Smith to fill in the blanks, the matrix would have looked like the matrix described in Table 10:2.

	% of individuals observing lions	% of individuals *not* observing lions
with Dr. Smith's Lion Powder	0%	100%
without Dr. Smith's Lion Powder	0%	100%

Table 10:2.   Likely outcome of a test of the effectiveness of Dr. Smith's lion powder.

You can see in an instant that Dr. Smith's powder is worthless, because the outcome doesn't change whether the powder is used or whether the powder is not used. The entries in the top row (from left to right) are in fact identical to the entries in the bottom row (from left to right). Hence, the outcome with or without Dr. Smith's Lion Powder remains unchanged. If you wanted to show mathematically that Dr. Smith's powder was worthless you would conduct a statistical analysis of the results given above and you would compute a number value called *a level of confidence* which can be attributed to the statement, "Dr. Smith's Lion Powder is effective." It is clear then that the level of confidence associated with this statement is in fact zero. In other words, the probability that Dr. Smith's Lion Powder is effective based upon the data derived from this "experiment" is zero percent. This matrix or tabular formulation is the essence of something called a *syllogism* developed by the ancient Greeks over 2,500 years ago and given mathematical or statistical meaning during the 18th and 19th centuries. We need not concern ourselves with statistics here. You may think of this matrix as a type of *truth matrix* if you will. The way in which the numbers fill in the matrix will tell you if the statement you are dealing with makes sense or is nonsense. As you will see later, some statements lie somewhere between complete sense and complete nonsense. A statement which is completely truthful is one to which we may attribute a 100% level of confidence. A statement which is completely nonsensical is a statement to which we may attribute a 0% level of confidence.

There is also another way in which the numbers or entries in a truth matrix can configure themselves so that the level of confidence is still low or zero. Let's assume that the young man was found sprinkling Dr. Smith's Lion Powder somewhere on the African plain or on a game preserve in an attempt to get rid of lions. The matrix would look like the matrix described in Table 10:3.

In this case, as in the previous case it is clear that it makes no difference whether the young man sprinkles the powder or not, the outcome is always the same. Still you might say, "What does all this lead to?"

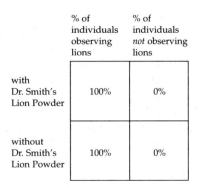

	% of individuals observing lions	% of individuals *not* observing lions
with Dr. Smith's Lion Powder	100%	0%
without Dr. Smith's Lion Powder	100%	0%

Table 10:3.   Likely outcome of a test of the effectiveness of Dr. Smith's Lion Powder in keeping lions out of an African game preserve.

Let me tell you of a true story more to the point. After sustaining a lower back injury I went to a chiropractor. He told me that I had scoliosis (a deformity of the spine) and that my injury had worsened that condition. He even showed me an X-ray of my spine illustrating deviant curvature in my spine. What more could I ask for, I had *real, tangible* proof in black and white. Only a fool would not believe his eyes, right? Well I unintentionally embarrassed the doctor when I asked him the following questions:

1. What percent of any given population having scoliosis as severe as mine has symptoms similar to mine?

2. What percent of any given population having scoliosis as severe as mine has *no* symptoms at all or is asymptomatic?

3. What percent of any given population *not* having scoliosis has symptoms similar to my own?

4. What percent of any given population *not* having scoliosis has *no* symptoms at all or is asymptomatic?

Sound familiar?

The doctor became visibly nervous. He admitted that during his 25 years of practice no one had ever asked him those questions.

At any rate, he told me what he would do in terms of manipulating my spine. That didn't stop me. I then asked him another set of questions:

1. How many people with my condition had recovered as a result of his treatment?

2. How many people with my condition had *not* recovered as a result of his treatment?

3. How many people with my condition had recovered by doing *nothing*?

4. How many people with my condition had *not* recovered by doing *nothing*?

5. How did he define the term, "recovered."

Sound familiar?

By now he was really nervous. I am not a sadist. I don't always enjoy putting people on the spot, but I had to know since my health and my money were at stake. To make a long story short, he didn't have any conclusive answers. The logical person would have run (if possible) and not walked out of his office. The illogical or the desperate person would have stayed.

This true story is not meant to put chiropractic medicine/therapy on the spot. It is meant only to illustrate a point I am making. I hope you now see what I'm driving at. The *syllogism* if appropriately applied can be extraordinarily powerful and revealing. Can you imagine what would occur if everyone asked his or her health care practitioner these questions every time a drug, diet, operation, or procedure were recommended? The situation would be quite dramatic. I suspect that a significant percentage of the health care establishment would undergo a major reorganization.

What would a truth matrix look like for a highly successful procedure or therapy? Let's call it Therapy X. In the extreme it might look something like the matrix in Table 10:4. The truth matrix for a highly unsuccessful treatment, Therapy Y, might look something like the matrix in Table 10:5.

	% recovered	% not recovered
with Therapy "X"	100%	0%
without Therapy "X"	0%	100%

Table 10:4.   Outcome of a test of Therapy "X" if that therapy were 100% successful.

	% recovered	% not recovered
with Therapy "X"	10%	90%
without Therapy "X"	50%	50%

Table 10:5.   Outcome of a test of Therapy "Y" if that therapy were not successful.

	% recovered or improved	% not recovered
In BioBalance	90%	10%
Out of BioBalance	0%	100%

Table 10:6. The outcome of BioBalance Therapy.

The matrix in Table 10:4 tells you that the Therapy X works whereas the matrix in Table 10:5 tells you Therapy Y does not work. In fact, in the latter case, the matrix tells you Therapy Y is downright dangerous in that it is worse than no therapy at all. Recall, Dr. Smith's Lion Powder was worthless. Therapy Y on the other hand is less than worthless, it is detrimental. There is a 50/50 chance of your recovering if you do nothing but only a 10% chance of your recovering if you engage in Therapy Y. A truth matrix of this nature can therefore give you an idea as to whether you should go ahead with a particular treatment as opposed to a competing treatment or no treatment at all. Table 10:6 provides an overview of the effectiveness of BioBalance Therapy.

I would now like to address another question I asked the chiropractor during my session with him, namely what is meant by the phrase "getting well"? You may feel that this question is silly, but if you think about it, it's not. Most people think you're well or you're not well. It turns out that there are scales of "wellness" which can be used to quantify how well you feel. These scales are important if any statement you make regarding biochemistry on the one hand and psychological and physical wellness on the other hand are to make any objective sense. If you want to know more about this, review my article published in the *International Journal of Biosocial Research* (see references). It is not necessary to discuss this in any detail here. I should point out that any measure of wellness should be replicable by anyone who wants to test or verify a mode of therapy. That is, a well structured experiment should be capable of being successfully repeated any number of times. A good measure of wellness should also indicate how long recovery lasts, if relapse occurs, as well as what percentage of a patient population actually gets worse. What good will a therapy, any therapy, be to you even if it is 100% successful, if you will relapse and possibly feel worse within a relatively short time after you're doing better. Clearly, high potency psychopharmacological agents can have you feeling absolutely fantastic and out of this world in no time flat. There's only one problem... they're addicting. None of these considerations is trivial.

As I have already shown you, BioBalancing routinely receives individuals failed by other types of dietary therapy. Given my knowledge of BioBalancing and acid/alkaline metabolism and biochemistry, it is my belief that these individuals comprise only a small percentage of those individuals who have been failed by various dietary therapies. If you were to subject each dietary therapy to the testing I have outlined above, as I have done, you would come up with the results I have listed in Chapter 4.

Still, you may persist in asking, *"But aren't you really like everyone else in telling people, believe me but don't believe anyone else?"* I have tried to show you how you can set up certain criteria to separate truths from half-truths and fictions. I am not asking you or telling you to believe in me. I am reporting published findings. BioBalancing has successfully assisted approximately 90% of candidate cases. By comparison the anecdotal success rates of other forms of nutritional therapy are lower than BioBalancing. Psychotherapy simply doesn't do any more good for you than a good heart-to-heart talk with a confidant. These are not opinions, they are based upon a statistically significant number of controlled observations.

Americans are spending *hundreds of billions of dollars* each year on medical care. To make matters worse, this enormous expense is rapidly escalating. With a ballooning national debt and ballooning twin deficits, Americans can ill afford this expense. In the event the future brings an economic recession (or worse still, a depression), that crisis will surely precipitate a national health care catastrophe. While I don't advocate an overthrow of the existing health care system, I feel that a major overhaul is long overdue. When three out of four individuals fall through the system's cracks and are thrown onto that system's administrative trash heap, namely psychotherapy, it is clear that there is something desperately wrong with primary health care. We need a cost effective alternative now. I submit that BioBalancing must form the foundation of that alternative.

Appendix

(Methods used to determine this information were published in
International Journal Biosocial Research, 1987: 9(2); 182-202.)

NUTRITIONAL REGIMEN APPROPRIATE FOR ACIDIC BIOCHEMICAL TYPES

RECOMMENDATIONS

Meat, Fish, Poultry:

ALLOWED: Organ meats such as liver, kidneys, brains, sweet-breads, tongue, tripe, etc.; pork ribs, bacon (*); all red meats including venison and veal†; lamb; cold cuts (*) of any variety but preferably additive-free; dark meat poultry (either chicken or turkey) such as poultry wings, thighs and drumsticks, skin may be left on when fried as desired (see methods of preparation below); duck and goose; all darker meat fish and some cold water fish either fresh, frozen or canned (*) such as salmon, dark meat tuna (often labeled as "chunk light") especially when packed in oil, swordfish, dark meat bluefish, mackerel, sardines (*), herrings (*), caviar and salmon roe, all shell fish such as scallops, abalone, oysters, clams and black mussels; escargot/snails; all crustaceans such as shrimp, crab, lobster and crayfish; squid/calamari, octopus; all frankfurters of any variety but preferably additive-free, including chicken franks, beef franks, pork franks, turkey franks and soy/tofu franks (see vegetables below).

AVOID: All light fish (either fresh or frozen) such as scrod, cod, flounder, sole, turbot, perch, haddock and fancy or solid white albacore tuna (*); chicken and turkey breast; lean pork, ham(*).

* All asterisked items are candida inducing.

† I would advise against eating veal for humane reasons.

MEAT, FISH AND POULTRY OF THE ALLOWED VARIETIES SHOULD BE EATEN AT EVERY MEAL. ABSTENTION FROM ALLOWED MEAT, FISH AND POULTRY WILL ACCENTUATE THE UNDERLYING ACIDIC STATE.

Vegetables:

ALLOWED: All leguminous vegetables such as peas, lentils and beans of any variety including tofu (soy bean curd), potatoes especially if fried or buttered to taste (fats will be discussed below), carrots, celery, spinach, cauliflower, artichokes as well as artichoke hearts (artichoke hearts bottled in oil are acceptable) and asparagus. All produce should be fresh and well rinsed to reduce pesticide ingestion. Individuals harboring significant levels of candida may at times be sensitive to insecticides used in agricultural application. Frozen produce may be used occasionally. It is suggested that canned produce (*) be avoided if possible. All gourd/autumnal squashes (*) such as Hokkaido pumpkin, buttercup squash, butternut squash and acorn squash may be eaten sparingly.

AVOID: Lettuce (any variety), tomatoes (any variety), cucumbers, peppers (any variety, sweet or hot), fresh garlic (garlic salt may be used sparingly), horseradish, onions (any variety) including leeks and scallions, cabbage of any variety, broccoli, broccoli raabe, mustard greens, eggplant, brussel sprouts, bean sprouts, zucchini and summer squash, kale, beets (*), sweet potatoes (*) and yams (*).

Fungi

ALLOWED: All mushrooms (*).

Fruits:

ALLOWED: Avocados and olives. Bananas may be used sparingly as a dessert or part of a meal. No more than 2 or 3 bananas should be consumed weekly. All bananas should be "green tipped" and not fermented to the point of being extremely ripe. The following fruits may be eaten cored and peeled, *sparingly* if desired and preferably with some nut or seed butter or at the end of an appropriate meal: apples and pears.

AVOID: All melons and citrus fruit (whether fresh or from concentrate) such as oranges, tangerines, grapefruits, lemons, limes, pineapple and tangelos. Also all of the following should be avoided as well: plums, apricots, peaches, berries, cherries and grapes.

Dairy:

ALL DAIRY SHOULD BE USED SPARINGLY AND NOT AS A PROTEIN SUBSTITUTE FOR MEAT, FISH OR POULTRY.

ALLOWED: Any whole dairy or cheese whether it be made from cow's milk or goat's milk; half n' half, heavy cream. If a lactose intolerance exists all dairy should be lactose reduced or if unavailable in this form, should be pretreated with *Lactaid*. This intolerance may not be an issue once BioBalance is achieved.

AVOID: Any dairy whose fat content is less than or equal to 2%.

Eggs:

ALLOWED: (either fertilized or unfertilized). Eggs may be prepared in any fashion. As is the case with whole dairy, eggs should not be regarded as a primary source of protein and as such should not be viewed as a substitute for meat, fish or poultry.

It must be emphasized that eggs and whole dairy may be used but should not be used as substitute for meat, fish or poultry of the allowed variety. To reemphasize a point made earlier regarding the relative importance of the allowed meats, fish and poultry, in the case of this particular regimen, *any meal lacking the allowed meats, fish or poultry is simply not a meal.*

Whole Grains:

ALLOWED: All whole grains. Whole grains include; brown rice (any length), whole barley, oats, buckwheat, corn, millet, rye, wheat and amaranth. Essene (*phon*. Ah-Seen) bread and rice cakes are primary choices among breads in that they contain neither flour or yeast. Essene breads or rice cakes with nut and/or seed butters make excellent snacks. Because of the acidic individual's excessively acidic condition, he or she should be discouraged from eating breads even though they may be of the primary variety unless those breads are used in moderation and accompanied by allowed meats, fish or poultry or with some combination of nuts, seeds, nut butters or seed butters (see below). Unleavened breads containing flour are also permitted but should be used *sparingly*, such as Norwegian flat bread, matzoh bread and sourdough bread. All other breads should be used very sparingly and avoided if possible regardless of the fact that they may be designated by the manufacturer as being "all natural," "whole grain," "organic," etc. Hot whole grains typically regarded as breakfast cereals such as buckwheat and oats may be eaten for breakfast but only in conjunction with allowed meat, fish and poultry. WHOLE GRAINS SHOULD BE EATEN DAILY AS A SIDE DISH for at least one meal per day to assist in maintaining normal bowel function.

AVOID: Any processed breakfast cereal (whether sugar free or otherwise) either hot or cold such as cream of wheat, wheatena, oat meal except as permitted above, rice krispies, puffed wheat, corn flakes, etc.

Nuts and Nut Butters:

ALLOWED: All nuts, peanuts (*) and seeds as well as nut and seed butters.

AVOID: None.

Fats:

ALLOWED: Olive oil, butter and lard. Corn or safflower oil may be used in stir frying.

AVOID: Safflower or corn oil (as a major source of fat); safflower, corn or soy margarine; mayonnaise.

Beverages:

ALLOWED: Decaffeinated coffee and tea. Weak, dilute tea. Weak, dilute fruit juice provided that it is not made from concentrate and provided that it is not of citrus extract may be used *sparingly*. For example, weak dilute whole apple juice is permitted. Club sodas and mineral waters are permitted as is distilled water.

AVOID: Soft drinks and alcoholic beverages. Coffee (nondecaffeinated), tea (nondecaffeinated) and all fruit juices with the exception of whole dilute noncitrus juice. Tap water may be used for cooking purposes unless there is reason to believe that its source is contaminated.

Miscellaneous:

ALLOWED: Salt to taste; fresh made meat and poultry gravies of any variety, rich fresh made poultry or beef stock (not all the fat should be skimmed); meat and poultry stock prepared in this fashion makes an excellent snack. Creamy based sauces and soups made with whole milk, half n' half or heavy cream (such as New England Clam Chowder). Shoyu, miso, tamari and soy sauce(*) are permitted.

AVOID: Lean, dilute, clarified chicken broth (irrespective of the type of meat (light or dark) used in preparing the broth) may be used *sparingly* and not as a main source of sustenance; dehydrated bullion cubes, monosodium glutamate, mustard, ketchup, horse radish, hot sauce, mayonnaise, salad dressing, fresh or powdered garlic and vinegar. Tomato based sauces and soups. As a rule, processed foods and "party" foods should be avoided or used very sparingly.

Desserts:

ALLOWED: Subject to the warning that all desserts should be used *very sparingly* if not avoided until candida overgrowth is brought under control, the following desserts are allowed; Ice cream, cheese cake, pastries, etc. Fruit of the appropriate variety is always permitted but *only* if used *sparingly* in conjunction with an allowed meal or with nut/seed butters.

AVOID: Zero or low fat sherbet such as Sorbet (*Phon*. Sor-Bay), fruit pies and torts.

A NOTE ON RESTAURANT DINING

While fast-food dining is not encouraged, eating high protein (ie. *meat*) fast-food fare in event of an emergency is not without merit in that it is more advantageous in this case to eat fast food when nothing else is available than to go without food for prolonged periods of time and incur the risk of becoming excessively acidic. In any event, planning ahead is the rule that should be observed. Standard fast food fare such as hamburger (without the bun and without condiments) and french fries (without condiments) is acceptable in event of an emergency.

METHODS OF PREPARATION

Any method of preparation is acceptable. Saute and stir fry are encouraged.

While any method of whole grain preparation is acceptable, some basic methods of preparing whole grains are summarized below:

Brown Rice or Barley: Add 3 cups of either grain to 5 cups of water in a stainless steel pressure cooker. Bring to full head of steam, reduce heat to low, insert a heat deflector element between the pressure cooker and the heating element (gas or electric) and let cook for 50 minutes.

Buckwheat or Millet: Any desired amount of either grain may be pan toasted over low heat in a cast iron skillet for 10 to 15 minutes, stirring occasionally. An equal amount of water or more if desired should then be added. Cover and let simmer until water is fully absorbed.

Typical Breakfast, Lunch and Dinner

BREAKFAST: Sausage link(s) (not spicy) with hash browned potatoes fried in small amount of residual sausage fat and/or butter. 1 cup of decaffeinated coffee (half n' half optional).

MID MORNING SNACK: (optional) 1 thin slice of Essene bread with any choice of nut butter.

LUNCH: Spinach salad with garbanzo beans, artichoke hearts and salmon. Dressing to consist of 1/4 wedge of fresh squeezed lemon, olive oil, salt to taste. 1 cup of herbal tea.

MID AFTERNOON SNACK: (optional) 1 cup of fresh made meat or poultry stock, or 1/4 apple with any choice of nut or seed butter.

DINNER: Cup of split pea soup, sauteed chicken liver (with small amount of sauteed onion), stir fried carrots, cauliflower and brown rice, 1 cup of herbal tea.

IT CANNOT BE TOO STRONGLY EMPHASIZED THAT INSOFAR AS THIS REGIMEN IS CONCERNED, ANY MEAL LACKING THE ALLOWED MEAT, FISH AND POULTRY IS LESS THAN ACCEPTABLE

Recommended Vitamin/Mineral Supplements

Supplements should *never* be taken until after an individual's acid/alkaline BioProfile has been well defined over a minimal period of 30 days. In the event these supplements cannot be tolerated, they should not be taken.

It is suggested that all vitamins be taken in hypoallergenic form. Experience suggests that the off-the-shelf brands "Solgar," "Twin Labs" and "KAL" produce predictable results. Other brands produce unpredictable results. Ideally all supplements should be taken sublingually in suspended solution. At the present time there is no known manufacturer which will produce the combinations of supplements required in this case in this particular fashion. A variation of 25% in dosage should not affect therapeutic outcome.

A full dose of vitamins is defined as follows:

Vitamin/Mineral	Full Dose
A (palmitate)	10,000 IUs
E (mixed tocopherols)	400 IUs
B12	100 mcgs
Niacinamide	100 mgs
Pantothenic Acid or Calcium Pantothenate	100 mgs
Inositol	250 mgs
Choline	250 mgs
Calcium	500 mgs
Phosphorous	250 mgs
Iodine (derived from kelp)	0.15 mgs
Zinc	10 mgs

All minerals should be "chelated." Iodine will likely not be found in chelated form. Kelp is commonly the supplemental form for iodine. Insofar as the dosages listed above are concerned, the "elemental" quantity specified on the bottle's label and *not* the chelated amount constitute a "Full Dose" Hence if (for example) the label lists that each tablet contains 100 mgs of zinc chelate which in turn contains 10 mgs of elemental zinc, one tablet will satisfy the requirements listed here.

A full dose may be taken after breakfast and again after lunch.

These dosages are appropriate for an individual whose weight ranges from 120 to 200 pounds. Individuals weighing less than 120 pounds should take only half the dosages listed here, while individuals weighing more than 200 pounds should take 1.5 times the dosages listed here.

It is noteworthy that cold weather accentuates an underlying acidic condition. Hence acidic types must be especially rigorous with their regimens during episodes of especially cold weather.

NUTRITIONAL REGIMEN APPROPRIATE
FOR <u>ALKALINE</u> BIOCHEMICAL TYPES

RECOMMENDATIONS

Meat, Fish, Poultry:

ALLOWED: All light fish (either fresh or frozen) such as scrod, cod, flounder, sole, turbot, perch, haddock and well rinsed fancy white albacore tuna packed in water (*); ideally white tuna should be soaked in water and refrigerated for at least twelve hours prior to consumption; as a rule of thumb with exceptions noted below, if the color of the fish in question is pure white or pale off-white then it is in all probability acceptable; lean, skinned chicken and turkey breast; lean pork, low salt ham (*) should be pretreated in the same fashion as tuna; low salt/low fat sausages may be eaten but not for breakfast. Meat, fish or poultry of any variety should NEVER be eaten for breakfast (a sample menu is listed below).

AVOID: Organ meats such as liver, kidneys, brains, sweetbreads, tongue, tripe, etc.; fatty pork, bacon (*) and heavily salted hams (*); all red meats including venison and veal; lamb; duck and goose; cold cuts of any variety (*); poultry wings, thighs and drumsticks; all darker meat and some cold water fish either fresh, frozen or canned (*) such as salmon, dark meat tuna (often labeled as "chunk light"), swordfish, dark meat bluefish, mackerel, sardines, herrings, caviar and salmon roe; all shell fish such as scallops, abalone, oysters, clams and black mussels; escargot/snails; all crustaceans such as shrimp, crab, lobster and crayfish; squid/calamari, octopus; all frankfurters of any variety irrespective of the fact they may be low in salt and additive-free and "all natural," including chicken franks, beef franks, pork franks, turkey franks and tofu franks (see vegetables below).

---

* All asterisked items are candida inducing.

Vegetables:

ALLOWED: Lettuce (any variety), tomatoes (any variety), cucumbers (peeled if waxed), peppers (any variety, sweet or hot), fresh garlic (not garlic salt), fresh horseradish (if in a jar then it should be a low or no salt variety), onions (any variety) including leeks and scallions, potatoes of any variety (but NOT fried), cabbage of any variety, broccoli, broccoli raabe, mustard greens, eggplant (but NOT fried or parmigiana), brussel sprouts, bean sprouts, zucchini and summer squash. Kale, sweet potatoes (*), yams (*), and all gourd/autumnal squashes (*) such as Hokkaido pumpkin, buttercup squash, butternut squash and acorn squash may be eaten in moderation. FRESH SALADS SHOULD BE EATEN DAILY. All produce should be fresh. Frozen produce may be used occasionally. It is suggested that canned produce (*) be avoided if possible. Celery and carrots should be used sparingly. Carrot shavings in a salad are appropriate whereas several carrots as part of a snack are inappropriate.

AVOID: All leguminous vegetables such as peas, beans and lentils of any variety including tofu (soy bean curd); spinach, cauliflower, artichokes and asparagus.

Fungi:

AVOID: all mushrooms (*).

Fruits:

ALLOWED: Any melon and fresh citrus fruit such as oranges, tangerines, grapefruits, lemons, limes, pineapple and tangelos, including fresh squeezed citrus juice (not from concentrate). Melons and fresh citrus or its juice should be eaten/drunk each morning (see outline of typical breakfast/lunch and dinner). While citrus may be eaten at any time of the day, the following fruits should be eaten in the afternoon only if desired: apples (peeled and cored), pears (peeled and cored), plums, apricots, peaches, berries, cherries and grapes. Except for extreme cases of candidiasis, fresh fruit is not candida inducing.

AVOID: Avocados and olives. Bananas may be used *sparingly* as a dessert or part of a meal (*never* for breakfast or in the a.m.). No more than 2 or 3 bananas should be consumed weekly. All bananas should be "green tipped" and not fermented to the point of being extremely ripe, black or moldy.

Dairy:

ALLOWED: Any dairy (cow's or goat's milk, yogurt and cottage cheese) whose fat content is less than or equal to 1.5%. If a lactose intolerance exists all dairy should be lactose reduced or if unavailable in this form, should be pretreated with Lactaid. This intolerance may not be an issue once BioBalance is achieved. Yogurt need not be pretreated. Low fat ricotta cheese and low fat mozzarella cheese are permitted in *small* quantities only during the evening meal if desired. Low fat ricotta and mozzarella should *never* be used as a main source of protein. Because of its salt content it is advisable that low fat mozzarella cheese be pretreated in the same fashion as tuna and ham (stated above). It is of course impossible to pretreat mozzarella cheese with lactaid and in this regard, this recommendation may be overlooked here.

AVOID: Any other dairy and cheese (*) whether or not it is lactose reduced. In essence, all dairy which contains 2% milk fat or more should be avoided.

Eggs:

ALLOWED: Eggs of any variety whether they are fertilized or unfertilized. Ideally, eggs should *not* be eaten for breakfast on a regular basis. They may be fried only with a small amount of margarine and *not* butter. Fats are discussed in additional detail below. Poaching or boiling are permitted.

Whole Grains:

ALLOWED: All whole grains with the exception of corn (see below). Whole grains include; brown rice (any length), oats/oat meal, whole barley, buckwheat, millet, rye, wheat and amaranth. The use of Essene (*phon*. Ah-Seen) bread and rice cakes is encouraged in that these breads contain neither flour or yeast. Unleavened breads containing flour are also permitted but should be used in moderation, such as Norwegian flat bread, matzoh bread and sourdough bread. All other breads (*) should be used sparingly if not avoided. Any sugar free breakfast cereal is also permitted such as corn flakes (despite the fact corn is not permitted), puffed rice, shredded wheat, cream of (brown) rice, cream of rye, etc. With the exception of Essene bread, rice cakes and breakfast cereals, whole grains should not be introduced until the afternoon and evening meals. Whole grains should be eaten daily.

AVOID: Corn and popcorn.

Nuts and Nut Butters:

AVOID: All nuts and seeds as well as nut and seed butters, especially peanuts and peanut butter.

Fats:

ALLOWED: Safflower or corn oil; safflower, corn or soy margarine; "all natural" sugar-free mayonnaise is preferable although other types of mayonnaise are permitted if used sparingly.

AVOID: Olive oil, butter and lard.

Beverages:

ALLOWED: Regular coffee (not decaffeinated) may be used "medicinally" in that caffeine is extremely acid inducing in its potential and may be used to abort an especially severe alkaline episode. One cup of regular coffee each morning with breakfast should be encouraged unless an idiopathic reaction occurs. In the unlikely event that such a reaction occurs, it will likely occur within the first few days of the program and consist of stomach cramps. An additional cup of coffee later in the day may also be drunk if needed, especially to counter-effect midafternoon fatigue. Regular tea (nondecaffeinated) may also be used instead of coffee. Tea however is less acid inducing than coffee and is more candida inciting in its potential than coffee. Low sodium or zero sodium club soda is permitted as is distilled water. Tap water may be used for cooking purposes unless there is reason to believe that its source is contaminated. While fruit juice concentrates(*) should ideally be avoided, they may be used sparingly (tomato juice and fruit juice). Fresh fruit juices, especially citrus fruit juices are encouraged. If diluted lemon or lime juice can be tolerated (not from concentrate or reconstituted), it may be used to abort alkaline episodes and achieve transient BioBalance.

Alkaline types must keep well hydrated, especially, but not exclusively in hot weather. It is noteworthy that hot weather will tend to accentuate an underlying alkaline imbalance. Consequently, alkaline types may want to abstain from eating all meat, fish and poultry, and possibly eggs during extreme hot weather spells, substituting low fat yogurt instead.

AVOID: Soft drinks and alcoholic beverages whose alcohol content does not exceed 12% by volume may be used *very sparingly*. Any alcoholic beverage whose content by volume exceeds 12% should be avoided, especially mixed drinks made with milk fat.

Miscellaneous:

ALLOWED: Lean, dilute, clarified chicken broth (irrespective of the type of meat (light or dark) used in preparing the broth); once again, meat or meat byproducts should *never* be eaten for breakfast; low or no salt, additive-free mustard, ketchup (*), horse radish, hot sauce, mayonnaise (*), salad dressing and vinegar (*) may be used. Tomato based sauces and soups are permitted provided that they are home made and provided that sauces do not contain excessive amounts of oil and salt, and do not contain any of the foods which should be avoided. Canned tomatoes (*) may be used on occasion. Low fat (1.5% or less) milk based soups and sauces may also be used if they are prepared with low fat lactose reduced milk, eggs, potato flour (not arrowroot or cornstarch) and any allowed oil or margarine so as not to exceed the individual's daily caloric fat intake. The absence of these soups and sauces could result in a rather boring cuisine and may prove discouraging. Any herb or spice may be used in moderation. Fresh garlic may also be used, generously if desired.

AVOID: Added salt, meat gravies of any variety, dehydrated bullion cubes, monosodium glutamate, creamy based sauces and soups made with whole milk, half n' half or heavy cream (such as New England Clam Chowder). As a rule, processed foods and "party" foods such as potato chips, tortilla chips, etc., should be avoided or used very sparingly irrespective of whether they are low in salt or not. Shoyu, miso, tamari and soy sauce should be used *very sparingly*.

Desserts:

ALLOWED: Subject to the warning that all desserts should be used *very sparingly*, the following desserts are allowed; zero or/low fat sherbet such as Sorbet (phon: Sor-Bay), fruit pies or torts absent the crust especially if the crust is high in fat and contains lard or butter. Fruit of the allowed variety is always permitted. In the event excessive alkalinity occurs which will result in the reemergence of pre-existing symptoms, a snack of citrus, accompanied (if desired) by low/no salt rice cakes and some nondecaffeinated coffee with a small amount of sugar may be ingested. The probability is rather high that within 30 to 60 minutes there will be a significant reduction in symptom severity.

In the case of the alkaline individual, sugar offers risks as well as benefits in that if taken sparingly it can have therapeutic effects since sugar is highly acid-inducing and will thus serve to reduce pre-existing alkaline imbalance which is the primary source of the distress in this case. Excessive ingestion of sugar however (more than approximately 1 to 2 level teaspoons per day) will serve to increase risk for incurring candida overgrowth.

Furthermore concentrated fats as incorporated in the desserts described below will produce deleterious effects which will far outweigh any of the transient benefits which may be derived by occasionally ingesting *small* amounts of sugar.

AVOID: Ice cream, cheese cake, pastries, etc.

A NOTE ON RESTAURANT DINING

Most restaurants offer an acceptable or allowed "catch of the day." Broiled or baked fish without fatty sauces that usually accompany seafood of this fashion is acceptable. Seafood fried in batter ("tempura") should be avoided. If appropriate seafood is not available, chicken breast or lean pork (in that order of preference) may be ordered. All "Fast Foods" should be avoided. If possible, low salt cuisine is always preferable. Salt should not be added. Currently, the product "Mrs. Dash's" may provide an alternative to salt. "K Salt" is not recommended.

METHODS OF PREPARATION

Any method is acceptable except for deep fat frying or tempura frying. To reiterate, fast foods are to be avoided. Stir frying is permitted if *small* amounts of allowed fat are used to lightly coat the wok or skillet to prevent sticking. Stir frying in this fashion should be encouraged in that it will add variety to what could easily become rather boring cuisine. It is suggested that aluminum cookware not be used. Stainless steel, cast iron, glass and ceramic are all acceptable. Teflon is also acceptable. Once again, ideally salt should not be added.

Some basic methods of preparing whole grains are summarized below:

Brown Rice or Barley: Add 3 cups of either grain to 5 cups of water in a stainless steel pressure cooker. Bring to full head of steam, reduce heat to low, insert a heat deflector element between the pressure cooker and the heating element (gas or electric) and let cook for 50 minutes.

Buckwheat or Millet: Any desired amount of either grain may be pan toasted over low heat in a cast iron skillet for 20 to 30 minutes, stirring occasionally. An equal amount of water or more if desired should then be added. Cover and let simmer until water is fully absorbed.

Typical Breakfast, Lunch and Dinner

BREAKFAST: 1 cup of regular coffee (freeze dried but not decaffeinated), 1 glass fresh squeezed orange juice, 1/2 grapefruit, 1 bowl of shredded wheat with low fat lactose reduced milk.
Meat, fish poultry and eggs should not be eaten for breakfast at any time.

MID MORNING SNACK: (optional) 1 cup of regular coffee (if desired) or weakly brewed tea plus 1 orange or tangerine.

LUNCH: Salad consisting of: Lettuce, tomatoes, radishes, onions, peppers, cucumbers (peeled if waxed), shredded cabbage, raw broccoli plus one or two hard boiled eggs. If eggs elicit an adverse reaction then they should be eliminated and coffee intake should be reduced in an attempt to avoid excessive acid induction. Salad dressing may consist of safflower oil, freshly squeezed lemon and minced garlic (if desired); 1 slice of Essene bread or rice cake(s). Beverage may consist of herbal tea (any variety) or weakly brewed regular tea.
Some alkaline types may wish to avoid meat, fish, poultry *and* eggs for lunch as well in the event some symptoms reemerge in the afternoon. In the event meat, fish, poultry and eggs are not included as part of lunch then low fat dairy (preferably low fat yogurt) should form the basis of protein intake during the morning and afternoon.

MID AFTERNOON SNACK: (optional) 1 cup of regular coffee (if desired) or weakly brewed tea plus 1 peeled, cored apple and tangerine.

DINNER: Fillet of Sole baked with lemon and teaspoon of safflower oil. Steamed zucchini and tomatoes, baked potato and brown rice. Safflower or corn oil or margarine may be placed on the vegetables and rice. 1 cup of herbal tea (any variety).

It must be re-emphasized that this is not a "high coffee" diet and that coffee should *never* be used indiscriminately and only "medicinally" as described above.

RECOMMENDED VITAMIN/MINERAL SUPPLEMENTS

Supplements should *never* be taken until after the individual's acid/alkaline BioProfile has been well defined over a minimal period of 30 days. In the event these supplements cannot be tolerated, they should not be taken.

It is suggested that all vitamins be taken in hypoallergenic form. Experience suggests that the off-the-shelf brands "Solgar," "Twin Labs" and "KAL" produce predictable results. Other brands produce unpredictable results. Ideally all supplements should be taken sublingually in suspended solution. At the present time there is no known manufacturer which will produce the combinations of supplements required in this case in this particular fashion. A variation of 25% in dosage should not affect therapeutic outcome.

A full dose of vitamins is defined as follows:

Vitamin/Mineral	Full Dose
A (fish liver oil)	10,000 IUs
D	400 IUs
C	500 mgs
B1	10 mgs
B2	10 mgs
B6	10 mgs
Niacin	25 mgs
Para Amino Benzoic Acid	100 mgs
Folic Acid	200 mcg
Biotin	150 mcg
Potassium	200 mgs
Magnesium	100 mgs
Iron	15 mgs
Copper	1 mg
Manganese	5 mgs
Chromium	100 mcg

All minerals should be "chelated." Insofar as the dosages listed above are concerned, the "elemental" quantity specified on the bottle's label and *not* the chelated amount constitute a "Full Dosage." Hence (for example) if the label lists that each tablet contains 500 mgs of magnesium chelate which in turn contains 100 mgs of elemental magnesium, one tablet will satisfy the requirements listed here.

A full dose is to be taken after breakfast and again after lunch. If an intolerable niacin "flushing" reaction occurs, then the dosage of niacin *only* is to be reduced to 10 mgs per full dose. Flushing is defined as similar to transient sunburn. It is noteworthy that the probability of occurrence of a "flushing" reaction at 25 mgs of Niacin per full dose is extremely low.

These dosages are appropriate for an individual whose weight ranges from 120 to 200 pounds. Individuals weighing less than 120 pounds should take only half the dosages listed here, while individuals weighing more than 200 pounds should take 1.5 times the dosages listed here.

It is noteworthy that hot weather accentuates an underlying alkaline condition. Hence alkaline types must be especially rigorous with their regimens during episodes of extremely hot weather. As indicated, alkaline types may wish to abstain from eating meat, fish and poultry as well as eggs in extremely hot weather, substituting only low fat dairy for protein.

While BioBalance Therapy makes no claims for dread disorders (terminal), casual observation of isolated cases suggests that to some extent these disorders may be *pH driven* as are the so-called psychogenic disorders. Accordingly, alkaline types suffering dread disorders may wish to consult with their physicians and modify the regimen described above by eliminating all meat, fish, poultry, eggs and dairy products with the exception of low fat yogurt. Low fat yogurt may be introduced in the midafternoon or evening as desired. In summary, this variation would consist of low fat yogurt, whole grains, (allowed) vegetables and (allowed) fruits. It is also important that these individuals have complete bowel evacuation daily. Consequently, in the event elimination is a problem, an enema or colonic should be administered daily until regular evacuation is achieved.

Nutritional Regimen Appropriate for Mixed Biochemical Types

This regimen divides foods into two categories, "Primary" and "Secondary." Mixed types should calorically mix the primaries with the secondaries in a 2:1 ratio at every meal. Hence, the regimen appropriate for normals lies somewhat closer to the regimen appropriate for acidics than the regimen appropriate for alkaline types. While tilting somewhat in favor of the primaries is a more forgiving error than tilting too far in favor of the secondaries, complete elimination of the secondaries from this regimen will cause the individual to become too alkaline and suffer accompanying distress.

Recommendations

Meat, Fish, Poultry:

PRIMARY: Organ meats such as liver, kidneys, brains, sweet-breads, tongue, tripe, etc.; pork ribs, bacon (*); all red meats including venison and veal†; lamb; cold cuts (*) of any variety but preferably additive-free; dark meat poultry (either chicken or turkey) such as poultry wings, thighs and drumsticks, skin may be left on when fried as desired (see methods of preparation below); duck and goose; all darker meat fish and some cold water fish either fresh, frozen or canned (*) such as salmon, dark meat tuna (often labeled as "chunk light") especially when packed in oil (*), swordfish, dark meat bluefish, mackerel, sardines (*), herrings (*), caviar and salmon roe, all shell fish such as scallops, abalone, oysters, clams and black mussels; escargot/snails; all crustaceans such as shrimp, crab, lobster and crayfish; squid/calamari, octopus; all frankfurters of any variety but preferably additive-free, including chicken franks, beef franks, pork franks, turkey franks and soy/tofu franks (see vegetables below).

SECONDARY: All light fish (either fresh or frozen) such as scrod, cod, flounder, sole, turbot, perch, haddock and fancy or solid white albacore tuna (*); chicken and turkey breast; lean pork, ham (*).

* All asterisked items are candida inducing.

† I would advise against eating veal for humane reasons

MEAT, FISH AND POULTRY OF THE PRIMARY VARIETIES SHOULD BE EATEN AT EVERY MEAL WITH THE OCCASIONAL EXCEPTION OF BREAKFAST. PROLONGED ABSTENTION FROM PRIMARY MEAT, FISH AND POULTRY WILL ACCENTUATE THE UNDERLYING ACIDIC COMPONENT OF THE MIXED METABOLIC STATE.

Vegetables:

PRIMARY: All leguminous vegetables such as peas, lentils and beans of any variety including tofu (soy bean curd), potatoes especially if fried or buttered to taste (fats will be discussed below), carrots, celery, spinach, cauliflower, artichokes as well as artichoke hearts (artichoke hearts bottled in oil are acceptable) and asparagus. All produce should be fresh and well rinsed to reduce pesticide ingestion. Individuals harboring significant levels of candida may at times be sensitive to insecticides used in agricultural application. Frozen produce may be used occasionally. It is suggested that canned produce (*) be avoided if possible.

SECONDARY: Lettuce (any variety), tomatoes (any variety), cucumbers, peppers (any variety, sweet or hot), fresh garlic (garlic salt may be used sparingly), horseradish, onions (any variety) including leeks and scallions, cabbage of any variety, broccoli, broccoli raabe, mustard greens, eggplant, brussel sprouts, bean sprouts, zucchini and summer squash, kale, beets (*), sweet potatoes (*), and yams (*), gourd/autumnal squashes (*) such as Hokkaido pumpkin, buttercup squash, butternut squash and acorn squash.

Fungi

PRIMARY: All mushrooms (*).

Fruits:

PRIMARY: Avocados and olives. Bananas may be used sparingly as a dessert or part of a meal. No more than 2 or 3 bananas should be consumed weekly. All bananas should be "green tipped" and not fermented to the point of being extremely ripe. The following fruits may be eaten cored and peeled, sparingly if desired and preferably with some nut or seed butter: apples and pears.

SECONDARY: All melons and citrus fruit (whether fresh or from concentrate) such as oranges, tangerines, grapefruits, lemons, limes, pineapple and tangelos. Also all of the following should be avoided as well: plums, apricots, peaches, berries, cherries and grapes.

Dairy:

ALL DAIRY SHOULD BE USED SPARINGLY AND NOT AS A PROTEIN SUBSTITUTE FOR MEAT, FISH OR POULTRY.

PRIMARY: Any whole dairy or cheese whether it be made from cow's milk or goat's milk; half n' half, heavy cream. If a lactose intolerance exists all dairy should preferably be lactose reduced or if unavailable in this form, should be pretreated with Lactaid. This intolerance may not be an issue once BioBalance is achieved.

SECONDARY: Any dairy whose fat content is less than or equal to 2%.

Eggs:

PRIMARY: (either fertilized or unfertilized). Eggs may be prepared in any fashion.

AS IS THE CASE WITH WHOLE DAIRY, EGGS SHOULD NOT BE REGARDED AS A PRIMARY SOURCE OF PROTEIN AND AS SUCH SHOULD NOT BE VIEWED AS A SUBSTITUTE FOR MEAT, FISH OR POULTRY.

Whole Grains:

PRIMARY: All whole grains. Whole grains include; brown rice (any length), whole barley, oats, buckwheat, corn, millet, rye, wheat and amaranth. Essene (*phon*. Ah-Seen) bread and rice cakes are primary choices among breads in that they contain neither flour or yeast. Essene breads or rice cakes with nut and/or seed butters make excellent snacks. Because excessive carbohydrate intake will accentuate a mixed metabolizer's acidic condition the patient should be discouraged from eating breads even though they may be of the primary variety unless those breads are used in moderation and accompanied by allowed meats, fish or poultry or with some combination of nuts, seeds, nut butters or seed butters (see below). Unleavened breads containing flour are also permitted but should be used sparingly, such as Norwegian flat bread, matzoh bread and sourdough bread. All other breads should be used very sparingly and avoided if possible regardless of the fact that they may be designated by the manufacturer as being "all natural," "whole grain," "organic," etc. Cooked whole grains typically regarded as breakfast cereals such as buckwheat and oats may be eaten for breakfast but only in conjunction with allowed meat, fish and poultry. *Whole grains should be eaten daily as a side dish* for at least one meal per day to assist in maintaining normal bowel function.

SECONDARY: Any processed breakfast cereal (whether sugar free or otherwise) either hot or cold such as cream of wheat, wheatena, oat meal except as permitted above, rice krispies, puffed wheat, corn flakes, etc.

Nuts and Nut Butters:

PRIMARY: All nuts and seeds as well as nut and seed butters.

Fats:

PRIMARY: Olive oil and butter. Corn or safflower oil may be used in stir frying.

SECONDARY: Safflower or corn oil (as a major source of fat); safflower, corn or soy margarine; mayonnaise.

Beverages:

PRIMARY: Decaffeinated coffee and tea. Weak, dilute tea. Weak, dilute fruit juice provided that it is not made from concentrate and provided that it is not of citrus extract. For example, weak dilute whole apple juice is permitted. Club sodas and mineral waters are permitted as is distilled water.

SECONDARY: Soft drinks and alcoholic beverages. Coffee (nondecaffeinated), tea (nondecaffeinated) and all fruit juices with the exception of whole dilute noncitrus juice. Tap water may be used for cooking purposes unless there is reason to believe that its source is contaminated.

Miscellaneous:

PRIMARY: Salt to taste; fresh made meat and poultry gravies of any variety, rich fresh made poultry or beef stock (not all the fat should be skimmed); meat and poultry stock prepared in this fashion makes an excellent snack. Creamy based sauces and soups made with whole milk, half n' half or heavy cream (such as New England Clam Chowder). Shoyu, miso, tamari and soy sauce(*) are permitted.

SECONDARY: Lean, dilute, clarified chicken broth (irrespective of the type of meat (light or dark) used in preparing the broth) should be used sparingly and not as a main source of sustenance; dehydrated bullion cubes, monosodium glutamate or msg, mustard, ketchup, horseradish, hot sauce, mayonnaise, salad dressing , fresh or dried garlic and vinegar. Tomato based sauces and soups. As a rule, processed foods and "party" foods should be avoided or used very sparingly if not avoided.

Desserts:

PRIMARY: Subject to the warning that all desserts should be used very sparingly if not avoided until candida overgrowth is brought under control, the following desserts are allowed; Ice cream, cheese cake, pastries, etc. Fruit of the appropriate variety is always permitted in conjunction with an allowed meal or with nut/seed butters.

SECONDARY: Zero or low fat sherbet such as Sorbet (phon: Sor-Bay), fruit pies and torts.

A NOTE ON RESTAURANT DINING

While fast-food dining is not encouraged, eating high protein (ie. meat) fast-food fare in event of an emergency is not without merit in that it is more advantageous in this case to eat fast food when nothing else is available than to go without food for prolonged periods of time and incur the risk of becoming excessively acidic. In any event, planning ahead is the rule. Standard fast food fare such as hamburger (without the bun and without condiments) and french fries (without condiments) is acceptable in event of an emergency.

METHODS OF PREPARATION

Any method of preparation is acceptable. Sauteing and stir frying are encouraged.

While any method of whole grain preparation is acceptable, some basic methods of preparing whole grains are summarized below:

Brown Rice or Barley: Add 3 cups of either grain to 5 cups of water in a stainless steel pressure cooker. Bring to full head of steam, reduce heat to low, insert a heat deflector element between the pressure cooker and the heating element (gas or electric) and let cook for 50 minutes.

Buckwheat or Millet: Any desired amount of either grain may be pan toasted over low heat in a cast iron skillet for 20 to 30 minutes, stirring occasionally. An equal amount of water or more if desired should then be added. Cover and let simmer until water is fully absorbed.

Typical Breakfast, Lunch and Dinner

BREAKFAST:

OPTION A: Low fat sausage link(s) with hash browned potatoes fried, 1 cup of regular coffee (2% milk optional).

OPTION B: Bowl/cup of oat meal with sliced apple and 2% or whole milk; egg(s) any style; 1 cup regular tea with either milk or lemon.

MID MORNING SNACK: (optional) 1 thin slice of Essene bread with small amount of any choice of nut butter.

LUNCH: Spinach salad with lettuce, cherry tomatoes, garbanzo beans, sweet peppers, artichoke hearts with dark and light meat chicken. Dressing to consist of 1/4 wedge of fresh squeezed lemon, olive oil, salt. 1 cup of herbal tea.

MID AFTERNOON SNACK: (optional) 1 cup of fresh made meat or poultry stock, or 1/4 apple.

DINNER: Cup of split pea soup, extra lean chopped sirloin with lightly sauteed onion, carrots, broccoli and brown rice, 1 cup of herbal tea.

IT CANNOT BE TOO STRONGLY EMPHASIZED THAT INSOFAR AS THIS REGIMEN IS CONCERNED, WHILE THE PRIMARY MEAT, FISH AND POULTRY ARE OPTIONAL FOR BREAKFAST, THIS IS NOT THE CASE WITH LUNCH AND DINNER. LUNCH AND DINNER MUST CONTAIN A PRIMARY/SECONDARY BLEND OF MEAT, FISH OR POULTRY.

Recommended Vitamin/Mineral Supplements

Supplements should never be taken until after the individual's acid/alkaline BioProfile has been well defined over a minimal period of 30 days. In the event these supplements cannot be tolerated, they should not be taken.

It is suggested that all vitamins be taken in hypoallergenic form. Experience in this case suggests that only the off-the-shelf brand "Solgar" produce predictable results. Other brands produce unpredictable results. Ideally all supplements should be taken sublingually in suspended solution. At the present time there is no known manufacturer which will produce the combinations of supplements required in this case in this particular fashion. A variation of 25% in dosage should not affect thera-peutic outcome.

A full dose of vitamins is defined as follows:

Vitamin/Mineral	Full Dose
CiPlex	1 Tablet
Vitamin E (mixed tocopherols)	200 I.U.s
Solamins	1.5 Tablets

A full dose may be taken after breakfast and again after lunch.

These dosages are appropriate for an individual whose weight ranges from 120 to 200 pounds. Individuals weighing less than 120 pounds should take only half the dosages listed here, while individuals weighing more than 200 pounds should take one and one half times the dosages listed here.

It is noteworthy that cold weather accentuates the acidic component of the mixed metabolic state. Hence mixed types must be especially rigorous with their regimens during cold weather spells.

A final note. It would be an error for an individual possessing a mixed metabolic state to exclude the "secondary" foods from this regimen. Exclusion of this nature will result in a regimen appropriate for acidic types. Supplementing the regimen appropriate for acidics with the supplements listed above will not offset the extreme alkaline inducing potential of a regimen skewed in such a fashion.

References/Bibliography

Aihara, H. *Acid/Alkaline*, Japan Publications Harper & Row, 1983

Aihara, H. *Basic Macrobiotics*, Japan Publications/Harper and Row, 1985

Atkins, R. *Dr. Atkins' Super Energy Diet*, Crown, 1977

Atkins, R. *Dr. Atkins' Nutrition Breakthrough*, Morrow, 1981

Berger, S. *Dr. Berger's Immune Power Diet*, NAL Books, 1985

Cheraskin, E. & Ringsdorf, W. *Psychodietetics*, Simon and Schuster, 1983

Crook, W. *The Yeast Connection*, Professional Books, 1984

Diamond, H. & Diamond, M. *Fit for Life*, Warner Books, 1985

Feingold, B. *Why Your Child is Hyperactive*, Random House, 1974

Hoffer, A. & Walker, M. *Orthomolecular Nutrition*, Keats, 1978

Kushi, M. *The Book of Macrobiotics*, Japan Publications Inc., 1977

Kushi, M. *The Cancer Prevention Diet*, St. Martin's Press, 1983

Kushi, M. *Diet for a Strong Heart*, St. Martin's Press, 1983

Mendelsohn, R. *MalPractice*, Contemporary Books, 1981

Mendelsohn, R. *Confessions of a Medical Heretic*, Contemporary Books, 1984

Muramoto, N. *Healing Ourselves*, Avon, 1973

Norris, R. & Sullivan, C. *PMS, Premenstrual Syndrome*, Rawson Associates, 1983

Ott, J.N. *Health and Light*, Simon & Schuster Inc., 1973

Ott, J.N. *Light, Radiation and You*, Devin Adair, 1982

Ott, J.N. Color and Light: Their Effects on Plants, Animals and People, Parts 1-5, *International Journal of Biosocial Research*, 1985-1989

Pritikin, N. *The Pritikin Promise*, Simon & Schuster, 1983

199

Randolf, T. & Moss, R. *An Alternative Approach to Allergies*, Harper & Row, 1980

Saxe, J. *The Blind Men and the Elephant* (ill. Galdone, P.), McGraw Hill, 1963

Truss, O. *The Missing Diagnosis*, pub. by author, 1983

Watson, G. Differences in Intermediary Metabolism in Mental Illness, *Psychology Reports*, 1965, 563-582, M2-V17

Watson, G. *Nutrition and Your Mind*, Harper & Row, 1972

Watson, G. *Personality Strength and Psychochemical Energy*, Harper & Row, 1979

Wiley, R. Biochemical Oscillations and the Development of Organization, *Journal of Biological Physics*, Vol. 10, 31-41, 1982

Wiley, R. The Effect of Acid/Alkaline Nutrition on Psychophysiological Function. *International Journal of Biosocial Research*, 1987: 9(2); 182-202.

Wurtman, J. *Managing Your Mind and Mood with Food*, Rawson Associates, 1986

Index

W

Y

Biography

Dr. Wiley holds a doctorate in biological physics from Kent State University, a master's degree in physics from the University of Pennsylvania, and a master's degree in psychology from Clark University.

While employed in other areas utilizing his expertise in mathematics and physics, his avocation for the better part of the last 20 years has consisted of assessing the impact of acid/alkaline nutrition upon human behavior and disease.

Dr. Wiley's consulting firm, BioBalance Services, grew out of his desire to put the many years of his scientific endeavors to use within the health care community — to make BioBalance Therapy directly accessible to the public. While continuing as an executive and consultant outside of the health care field, he has spent the last three years as the director of BioBalance Services, assisting physicians and other health care practitioners in assessing and successfully correcting their patients' metabolic imbalances.

Dr. Wiley has published scientific articles in the field of biological physics in professional journals. His book, *BioBalance*, is his first publication written specifically for the general public. It is his firm conviction that once the health care community and the general public become aware of the momentous impact of underlying metabolic imbalances on mental and physical health, proper blood pH evaluation will become as routine a part of any health examination as checking a patient's temperature or blood pressure.